Being Interprofessional

When I Heard the Learn'd Astronomer

When I heard the learn'd astronomer,
When the proofs, the figures, were ranged in columns before me,
When I was shown the charts and diagrams, to add, divide,
   and measure them,
When I sitting heard the astronomer where he lectured with
   much applause in the lecture-room,
How soon unaccountable I became tired and sick,
Till rising and gliding out I wander'd off by myself,
In the mystical moist night-air, and from time to time,
Look'd up in perfect silence at the stars.

Walt Whitman (1819–92)

Being
Interprofessional

Marilyn Hammick

Della Freeth

Jeanette Copperman

Danë Goodsman

polity

First published in 2009 by Polity Press

Polity Press
65 Bridge Street
Cambridge CB2 1UR, UK

Polity Press
350 Main Street
Malden, MA 02148, USA

ISBN-13: 978-0-7456-4305-2
ISBN-13: 978-0-7456-4306-9(pb)

A catalogue record for this book is available from the British Library.

Typeset in 10.5 on 13 pt Quadraat
by Servis Filmsetting Ltd, Stockport, Cheshire.
Printed in Italy by Rotolito Lobarda.

For further information on Polity, visit our website: www.politybooks.com

Contents

Illustrations

Figures

Photos

Tables

About the Authors

Professor Marilyn Hammick is an international Research and Education Consultant in health, social care and medical sciences. She is a Visiting Professor at Birmingham City University and Anglia Ruskin University, UK, Immediate Past Chair of the UK Centre for the Advancement of Interprofessional Education and Consultant to Best Evidence Medical Education. Her scholarly work focuses on evidence-informed education practice and policy, the translation of theory into practice and policy and the development, delivery and evaluation of interprofessional education. She is a member of the WHO Study Group on Interprofessional Education and Collaborative Practice and an associate editor of the *Journal of Interprofessional Care*. Marilyn practised as a radiographer at the Royal Marsden Hospital and other cancer care centres internationally.

Professor Della Freeth is Professor of Professional and Interprofessional Education at City University, London, and Head of the Education Development Unit within the School of Community and Health Sciences. She leads research and evaluation projects that focus on education designed to improve patient safety and the quality of care, particularly interprofessional education and learning through simulated professional practice. She is a member of the UK Centre for the Advancement of Interprofessional Education and served on its Board 1998–2005, and also co-convened the British Education Research Association special interest group 'Learning in the Professions' 2003–6. She is an associate editor of the *Journal of Interprofessional Care*.

Jeanette Copperman is a Senior Lecturer and Programme Director for Social Work, School of Community and Health Sciences, City University, London, teaching, researching and supervising research on interprofessional practice. She has experience as a community work practitioner in the voluntary sector and as a policy adviser in both local government and the health sector. Her past roles include Research Associate, Sainsbury Centre for Mental Health, and researching sexual violence with Barnardos' Policy Planning and Research Unit. She was an executive member of the Social Perspectives Network from 2004–8 and a specialist social care adviser to the UK Department of Health Victims of Violence and Abuse

Programme. Her research interests include gender issues, mental health and participatory research.

Dr Danë Goodsman is Senior Lecturer at Barts and the London School of Medicine and Dentistry, Queen Mary, University of London. She worked as a classroom teacher and lecturer in schools, colleges and universities. Her past roles include Curriculum Project Manager for the Royal College of Surgeons of England and Senior Lecturer and Education Adviser to Guy's, King's and St Thomas' Schools of Medicine and Dentistry. Her areas of interest are curriculum development and management, and teacher education and faculty development. Dr Goodsman has also been a member of the BMA's Board of Medical Education.

Acknowledgements

A book like this is written in the context of many professional and personal relationships and experiences. These informed its value base, shaped its content and provided inspiration for the practice of writing that such a task demands. Far too many people to list here provided all of that, and more, for us. We thank you all very much – and trust that you know who you are.

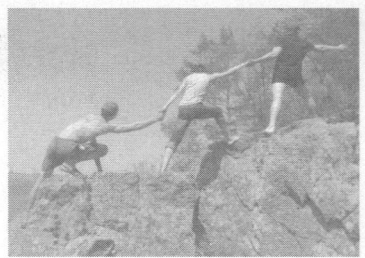

Introducing this book

This book was written for undergraduate students involved in interprofessional learning at UK universities, mainly those enrolled on programmes relevant to publicly funded services such as education, health care, social care and related subjects. We know, for example, that students of policing, law, criminal justice, housing and the built environment participate in interprofessional education. We welcome them as readers. In addition, newly qualified practitioners and postgraduate and continuing professional development learners will find the book relevant to their work and studies.

As we wrote this book, we kept our distinctive audiences and their range of interprofessional practice in mind. Interprofessional practice takes place where and when practitioners work collaboratively in order to meet service user and carer needs and expectations. It is challenging (and probably unhelpful) to put tight boundaries around the concept of interprofessional practice. At different times, different members of the workforce will work together. It is likely that the practice settings and organizations that employ these staff will also change, again, according to service need. The field is wide and constantly informed by emerging public service policies and priorities.

All of this gave us difficult choices about the book's content. We had to choose from the wide range of potential topics, their theoretical base and their application in service delivery settings. We needed to select with care the language and examples we used and be sensitive to the diverse politic across the subjects we touched on. In one sense we were spoilt for choice when it came to illustrating theory and issues. This meant we set aside some material that would have served the book well. We remain content with our choice to take the wide and long view.

Our readers will find that certain topics, most prominently communication, professionalism and children's services, are discussed in more than one place. On reflection, we recognize these as key narratives in the book: the first, because being interprofessional requires practitioners to also be professional; the second, because competency in communicating with others is a (some might argue, the) seminal requirement of being interprofessional. Children's services recur because of their current high profile and the lessons that the establishment of fit-for-purpose services for children and young people have for services delivered similarly to adults. We have 'joined up the dots' between the appearances of these by indicating cross-references in key places.

Our collaborative experience taught us that writing for an interprofessional audience has similar challenges and an equal complexity to interprofessional learning and working. Our reflection on our work is that a finer focus would have given us a simpler task, with more confidence that each and every one of our readers would find that everything in the book fits their professional and/ or personal frames of reference. However, this would have been to escape the essential nature of writing about being interprofessional and a diversion from what we wanted to do. We suspect that our readers will have to work hard to relate to and assimilate some of the content on a few of these pages. Your hard work is a worthwhile part of learning to be interprofessional and will be rewarding. Happy reading, learning and collaborative working to you all.

How the book is organized

The book is organized in three parts, each with its own introduction. Overall, the book takes you on a journey that begins with understanding the meaning of being interprofessional and why this way of being a professional practitioner is important. En route, it passes through many of the different places that require practitioners to work collaboratively and use their interprofessional knowledge and skills. Finally, it reaches the point where qualified practitioners step into the reality of practice. The book ends with a glossary and some information on interprofessional organizations.

Each part provides relevant material to support learning about others in the service delivery team, to enable you to learn from each other and to encourage learning with others to permit all perspectives, and possibly new perspectives, on practice to emerge. This learning and working team includes the client/patient/service user and unpaid carers.

Keeping a user focus to the work of the collaborative care team is a constant theme in the book. There are case studies of collaborative practice in a range of settings to help you identify with the realities of practice and to collaboratively engage with the professional and personal complexities as well as the delights and challenges of learning and working together. Learner exercises accompany much of the discussion. These are designed for you to do on your own and with others in the interprofessional team. At times you are encouraged to pause and reflect on what you have read. Our aim is for you to learn from this book and to actively engage with its content as a way of understanding what being interprofessional and working collaboratively mean.

Part I

Setting the Scene

In Part I we set down some of the things that we believe about being interprofessional. The opening chapter addresses the basic question we think our readers might ask on seeing the title of the book: what does being interprofessional mean? As the chapter progresses we first dissect the different parts of the title. Then we build a model to enable you to picture its meaning, as well as to read the story behind our proposition about what it means to be interprofessional.

Chapter 2 is our response to what would seem to be the reader's next question: why is being interprofessional important? This chapter also looks at the principles that underpin interprofessional learning and working.

We then turn to team-working: first, from the viewpoint of the individual team and its members, and, second, from a whole team and an organizational perspective. Chapter 3 confirms that interprofessional teams and their members have much in common with, and some differences from, other teams, and chapter 4 that organizations of many different hues have valuable roles to play in supporting and sustaining interprofessional practitioners.

1

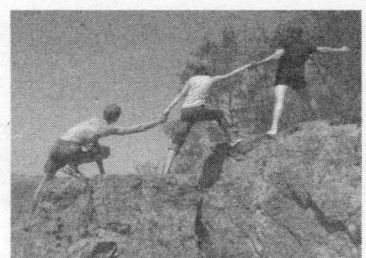

Being Interprofessional: Models and Meaning

We are what we believe we are.

C. S. Lewis

What you will read in this chapter

As its title indicates, this book is about *being interprofessional*. In this
first chapter we take the title apart and then put it back together again,
as a way of explaining what we mean by *being interprofessional*. In doing
this, we touch on the part that tradition plays in how staff in health and
social care settings and other related public services work together and
with the users of these services. We look at the knowledge, skills and
attitudes that contribute towards being a competent interprofessional
member of the service delivery team. Because being interprofessional
is related to your work, we've included a series of short case studies and
designed some learning exercises that relate to working in this way.

Being interprofessional: towards understanding

We hope you are reading this book because you are interested in
what being interprofessional means: whether you are a student or a
practitioner. That probably means you have some questions about being
interprofessional. Similarly, as we prepared to write this book, we had
our own questions about being interprofessional. Questions like:

What does it mean to be interprofessional?
What does being interprofessional involve?
When practitioners are interprofessional, how do they behave?

We use the word 'being' to indicate that what we are discussing concerns how we are, how we act and what we do in our professional and working lives. The word indicates that being interprofessional is always, or should always be, part of our professional lives. Ideally, being interprofessional is a routine and regular part of how we work, an active rather than passive practice-related behaviour. It is especially but not exclusively important in complex team working and multi-agency situations. It is not a way *to be* as a last resort or because a particular problem needs to be solved. Being interprofessional is only too often relegated to this 'only when things go wrong' status. You will read later how the consequences of not being interprofessional have often been very serious. Even with these lessons available to us, sometimes, even now, this key way of working is absent from many service delivery areas.

One way of looking at being interprofessional is to see it as involving thinking as well as feeling, and being able to take action (Figure 1.1). This makes being interprofessional rather complex. It means we have to orchestrate what we know, what we feel and what we can do, so that we behave in the right way.

So, *being interprofessional* means that we:

1. **Know what to do**: to *think* through what action is needed in a particular setting and how to do what is needed. This is often referred to as knowing the right thing to do.
2. **Have the skills to do** what needs to be done. This means being competent and capable of behaving and doing things correctly.

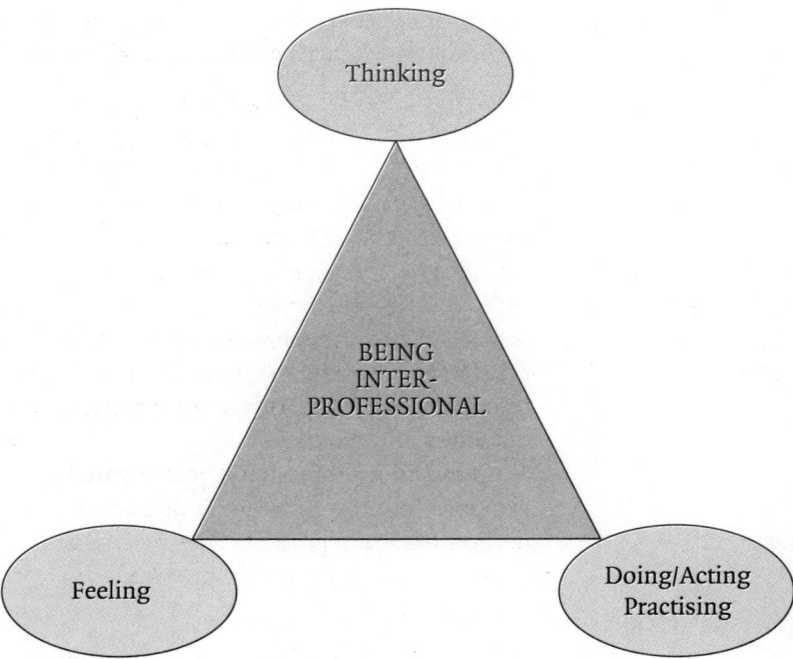

Figure 1.1 Three aspects of being interprofessional

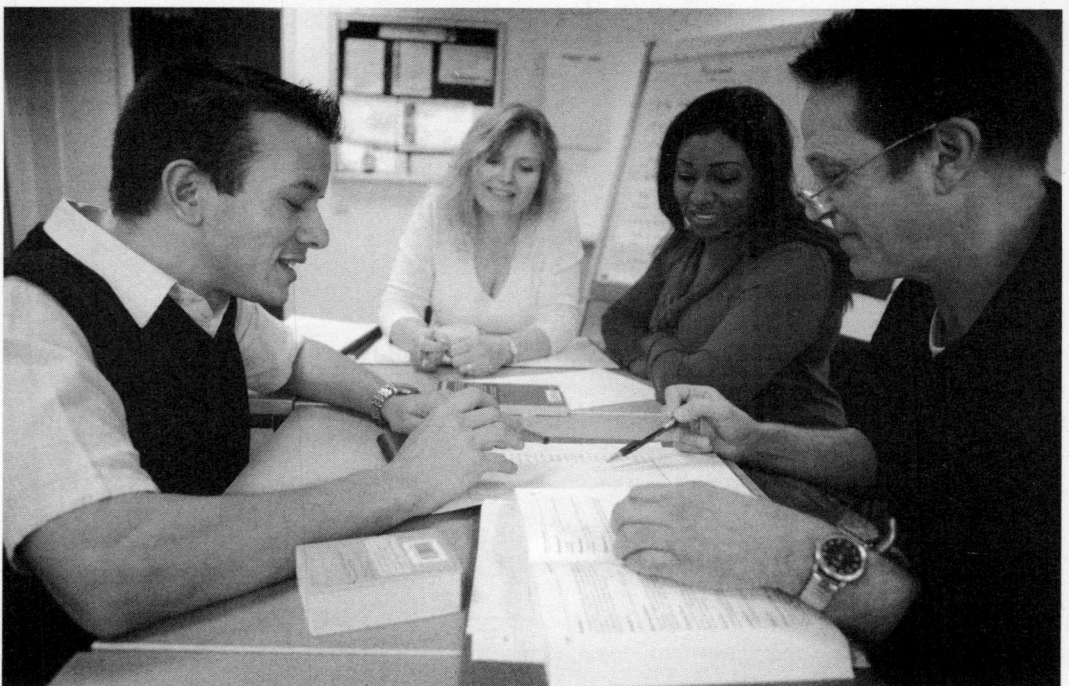

Photo 1.1 Being interprofessional begins as students and continues right through to managerial roles. Chris Schmidt/iStock.

3. **Conduct ourselves** in the right way when carrying out a particular action. This involves doing the task with the appropriate attitudes, and having suitable values and beliefs about what we are doing.

What any one of us needs to know, what skills we need and our attitudes will, of course, depend on our position and role in an organization. Being interprofessional as a student is different from practising in this way as a manager or advanced practitioner. Later on, we set out the knowledge, skills and attitudes we think are necessary for interprofessional competence for students leaving their initial education course to take up their first post (Box 1.4). But there are common features to the way all staff practise interprofessionally; again, we discuss these later. Here our aim is to understand what *being interprofessional* means, generally, for both ourselves and others.

Often 'interprofessional' is compared with other similar terms (for example, 'multiprofessional') that are close to it in meaning. These definitions are important. They mean that everyone reading and discussing these concepts understands what they mean. You will find examples of these for education and learning in the quotes below.

Interprofessional education occurs when learners from two or more professions learn about, from and with each other to enable effective collaboration and improve the quality of care. (Adapted from the original definition by the UK Centre for the Advancement of Interprofessional Education)

Interprofessional learning is learning arising from interaction between members (or students) of two or more professions. This may be a product of interprofessional education or happen spontaneously in the workplace or in education settings. (Hammick et al. 2007)

Multiprofessional education (MPE) is when members (or students) of two or more professions learn alongside one another: in other words, parallel rather than interactive learning. (Freeth et al. 2005)

Being interprofessional: towards a model

In the definitions of interprofessional education and interprofessional learning there are some clues to the characteristics or features of education and learning that make them interprofessional (Box 1.1).

We have used the clues in Box 1.1 to navigate a more complex and less travelled route towards a sense of knowing more about what being interprofessional is.

Being interprofessional

Being interprofessional is:

1   'Learning and working' or 'working and learning' with *others*: as appropriate, when necessary, and sometimes both: the important word here is **'and'**.

Box 1.1: Clues to the meaning of interprofessional

- Not something you do alone: it involves being with others/colleagues
- Not just for students: it is also for practitioners
- Not only planned: it can be spontaneous
- On the campus, in the classroom, in workplaces and workspaces
- The learning processes are not the *ends*: they are the *means* towards an end (or several ends)
- Education is characterized by learning about, learning from, and learning with others in order to add to what we already know
- Having an end implies there is a purpose: to improve collaboration, the quality of care and make gains in professional practice
- The focus on professional practice links the learning with working.

- Being interprofessional is being open to learning with the other people you work with, about that work, to improve (in every sense) the way you work
- Being interprofessional is, at the same time, working better together as the result of learning.

2 For everyone: learning and working, or working and learning with colleagues, is for everyone in any position.

- Being interprofessional applies at all stages of our working lives, from when we are beginning our professional careers to when we are in senior positions responsible for setting policy and leading organizations. Think about who you could possibly exclude from benefiting from the learning-working/ working – leaning pairs – we can't think of anyone!

3 Important, regardless of place and time, and applies in both routine and novel situations.

- It is possible to be interprofessional without knowing it: can you think of examples?

- It's also possible for the very team that needs to be interprofessional not to be working in this way.

4 Purposeful and has to be fit for that purpose.

- Being interprofessional is about collaborating in ways that are fit for purpose
- Being interprofessional is about collaboration as the means towards an end
- Being interprofessional is about improving practice/work/ service delivery.

Figure 1.2 summarizes some of the things that are helpful in knowing more about how to be interprofessional. Now we want to look closer at the importance of both parts of the word 'interprofessional': its stem (*inter*) and its root (*professional*).

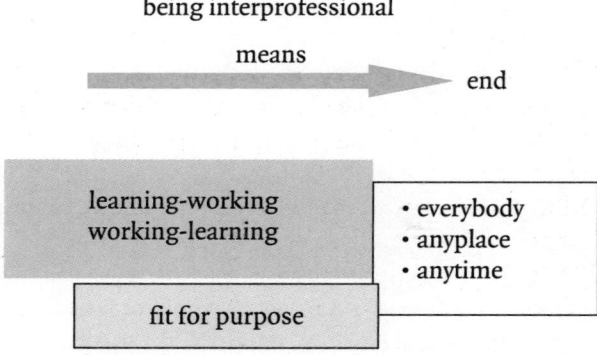

Figure 1.2 Being interprofessional: model A

The stem *inter* denotes a sense of between-ness, as shown by the words 'interstitial', 'interactive' and 'intermission'. Meanings for these are listed below and we've left a space for you to think of other words and their meanings that use *inter* as their stem.

An intermission is recognizable as that period of time between two acts of a play.
Your examples: inter. . .

When we speak of something as interactive we know it involves more than one person communicating or collaborating.
Your examples: inter. . .

The interstitial boundary between one type of body tissue and another can be identified microscopically.
Your examples: inter. . .

In our randomly chosen examples, *inter* indicates plurality or the involvement of more than one. All are associated with a space and time of their own, have their own presence and are independent of the entities that give rise to them. One of them, interstitial, indicates that a border or boundary is involved. What other meanings come to mind with your list of words using *inter*?

Remembering that our aim is to describe interprofessional in the same way as these other words, what does this brief focus on the stem of 'interprofessional' add to how we understand it? The picture of what it means to be interprofessional is developing (Figure 1.3). Now we can see that this way of being depends on more than one person, in a mutual space (virtual or real) and over a period of time, collaborating to bring their working and learning together. Importantly, for everyone involved, the means to the end (their mission, aim or purpose) is the same; and what they all do needs to be fit for purpose.

Two other things are worth noting in Figure 1.3. The working and learning of two people is similar, but it's not identical. Importantly, this emphasizes the value in the differences they bring to their joint working and the potential for these differences to contribute to a successful outcome. Many people make up an interprofessional team, including the users of services and their carers. The effective collaborative team is one where all members are working to the same purpose, with the aim that no gaps exist. The potential for two types of gap are highlighted below. There are others, some of which are particular to certain types of service delivery.

The first gap we want to say more about here results in the care or service provided being fragmented or, as is often described, not being 'seamless or joined-up'. Box 1.2 has some brief examples of people

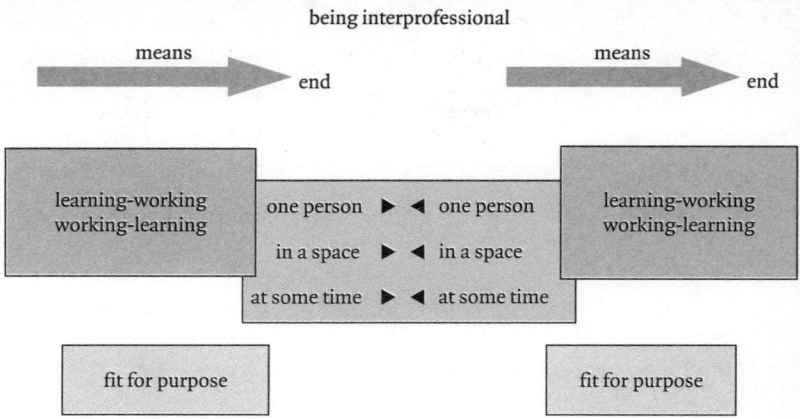

Figure 1.3 Being interprofessional: model B

who need joined-up care services; where practitioners need to work collaboratively if the needs of the service users and their carers are to be fully met. You will find more and extended examples later on in the book. For now, we want to give you a glimpse of the breadth of interprofessional working in today's health and human services. Learner Exercise 1.1 is designed with that in mind and can be done alone or as a group exercise.

Box 1.2: Examples where interprofessional working is necessary

Example 1

Bill lives with Jim and Sheryl, his son and daughter-in-law, following recent hip replacement surgery. Their house is small and everyone seems to get in each other's way. Several months ago, Sheryl tripped over Bill's walking frame so it's now kept outside. He fell the first time he tried getting to the toilet without it; Sheryl had to clean him up when she came home from shopping. At work, Jim has a call from the hospital to say that Bill is fine now and can be collected. When he arrives, the nurse asks to speak to him about the bruises on Bill's arms and legs . . .

Example 2

Kamilla is at home, recovering from surgery and radiotherapy to treat a malignant tumour on her tongue. She is being cared for by her parents and finds having visitors difficult. It is also difficult being back at her childhood home again after many years of independence. She knows that her mum and dad are finding the physical work of caring for her hard, and they aren't coping with her illness and disfigurement. She has a lot of pain and finds it difficult to swallow the tablets prescribed by the oncologist. Kamilla wonders if her medication comes as a liquid and if there is anyone else who has been in this position . . .

Example 3

Lucy has looked after her dad since her mum left the family home. At first she got to school on time, but now she often misses the bus. Lucy has many problems because her school doesn't understand her home life. If she is late she gets her dad to write a note saying that she was sick; he does this when she stays at home to let the community psychiatric nurse in. That happens when the nurse can't come after school. Lucy has tried not being there for the nurse, but Dad hides when he hears the doorbell. Lucy knows how important the nurse's visits are: Dad might have to go away if the nurse doesn't see him regularly. This happened once before and Lucy had to stay with relatives for a few days. Lucy worries about her dad when she is out, but would really like to go to town with her friends sometimes . . .

Example 4

Ahmad, Monique and their family had to leave their home very quickly the evening of the 2008 summer floods. They spend the next few days in the emergency shelter at a local school, grateful for the meals and the staff who keep the children occupied. There is an advice desk, so Ahmad finds out about insurance claims and temporary housing. Their third child is due in six weeks and Monique is very concerned about whether she could still have her baby at home. Ahmad has learnt that the clean water supply to their street was damaged and that in some houses the flood water has not yet receded. Ahmad and Monique wait to hear more about their house and their future . . .

Example 5

Alex, who is partially sighted, has just had his nineteenth birthday and, like all young people, feels it's time for him to find somewhere of his own to live. He also has learning disabilities which means that he needs a lot of attention, and he becomes very agitated in strange places. Jacqui, his mum, has always looked after him, and she would like him to stay at home and go to a day centre. Michael, his dad, thinks differently. He was recently diagnosed with coronary artery disease and has been advised to stop smoking and lose weight. It's difficult for Michael to cope with Alex's behaviour without a cigarette. Last week Alex stayed overnight in a house where other young people like him live. He enjoyed his stay but Jacqui has persuaded him that he wouldn't be happy there all the time. This week Alex and his family are meeting his support team to make some decisions . . .

From the work you have done for Learner Exercise 1.1, you have probably realized that a lack of joined-up care can happen for many reasons. Two of the most common are listed on the left side of Learner Exercise 1.2. The right side is blank for you to note why

Learner Exercise 1.1: Practitioners and staff who work interprofessionally

After reading the examples in Box 1.2, make a list of:

1 All the practitioners and staff who would have been involved in providing services to the person and their family in each example.
2 Practitioners and staff who might be involved with them in the future.

Is there anyone on the second list who would not be there if the first interprofessional team had been more inclusive?
How might the lives of the people in each example been different?

If you can, discuss your answers to these questions in an interprofessional learning team. This could be in a face-to-face group or using e-learning facilities. Think about what you know after the discussion that you didn't know before.

Learner Exercise 1.2: Identifying why there are gaps in the services provided to users

Reasons why services are fragmented or not joined-up	And the reason for this is. . .
The person who knew about this through their work or professional knowledge was not part of this cross-boundary collaboration.	
The needs of the service-user and their carer were not properly recognized.	

these things might happen. Read Box 1.2 again if you need some practice examples to help your thinking. We suggest that you do this exercise by yourself first of all: it should only take ten minutes. Then, if you can, do it with other students in the interprofessional team, perhaps when you are studying a classroom-based interprofessional module. If you are on a practice placement and can find one or more students from other professions, have a go with them. Try to note any differences between the reasons you gave when you did the exercise by yourself and the ones you gave when you did the exercise as part of an interprofessional student group.

Another gap at the interprofessional boundary appears between what one person does and says and what others hear and then do, or sometimes, what they then don't do. The death of Victoria Climbié highlighted the consequences of gaps between what was said and heard and not done (Laming 2003). We comment more on this later in this book.

Now we can see that communicating so that there is no gap includes:

1. Using language that everyone in the interprofessional team understands: steps towards this include watching out for jargon and not using acronyms. Often we just don't realize how much jargon and how many acronyms are in our working vocabulary. Take a moment to look at Pause Point 1.1 below: if you have time, discuss your list with someone from another profession. Make a note (this can be in your head) about how you might now change the way you communicate at work with others.

2. Taking time to listen to the meaning of what others are saying; rather than just hearing the words. This principle also applies to written communication: skimming the surface instead of reading with care might mean that you miss an essential element of what someone wants you to know. Ask yourself if you find the time and space to read with care and if you write in a way that others can understand. These days, with computerized record-keeping, understanding is less about deciphering a colleague's handwriting and much more about knowing what they wanted you to know from what they have written. Good record-keeping means recording what you observe, your telephone calls and details of face-to-face conversations, as well as keeping important email messages secure and retrievable.

3. Being aware of the importance of non-verbal communication and, for example, its role in conveying trust between people (Giddens 2006). The meaning of what we say is conveyed not only by our choice of words but also by facial expression and bodily gestures. These influence our understanding of what a colleague says to us

Pause point 1.1: Jargon and Acronyms

Jot down some of the jargon words and some acronyms you use as part of your job.

Look at each item on your list and decide:

- Whether a service user would know what it means
- If a colleague from another profession would understand what I meant if I said or wrote this.

See if you can match the items on your list with words that are from a language we can all share.

in a face-to-face conversation. It can be difficult to build effective interprofessional relationships when interaction is just via email and the phone. Can you think of times when it would have been better to have had a meeting with a colleague rather then send a message or make a call?

Being interprofessional: values and competencies

From the discussion so far we can conclude that, amongst other things, being interprofessional means:

- Being a willing and skilful communicator with others in the team, or in other teams and agencies; and
- Being aware of the knowledge and skills of your colleagues, and recognizing who can best meet the needs of a particular client.

Both these are included in the list of first-post interprofessional competences in Box 1.4, but a list of competences is incomplete without an indication of how these should be conducted. To understand more about this, we turn to the last part of our title and look at what *professional* contributes to the meaning of interprofessional.

You may have already had discussions with students from your own profession about what it means to be professional. This probably included looking at your relationship with the users of the services you offer, the general public and with each other. It is more likely to have involved issues such as client confidentiality and anonymity, and sharing information within your agency, rather than crossing boundaries and attitudes to other professionals (Jha et al. 2007). Later, in chapter 9, we discuss sharing information in interprofessional working in more detail.

In this section we focus on what it means to be professional in relation to knowing how to act interprofessionally with colleagues from different professions, and between practitioners who may not necessarily regard themselves as being part of a profession. Examples of these are people who provide transport and escort services for people with a disability, those who clean clinics and classrooms, and staff who are responsible for appointments in public service settings. In this respect we are using the word 'professional' to denote how someone behaves rather than to signal they belong to a group that practises in a certain way.

A profession is much wider than people may at first think, and being interprofessional includes working with all the people you come into contact with and who have an effect on patients or clients. The word 'profession' is generally used to describe a group

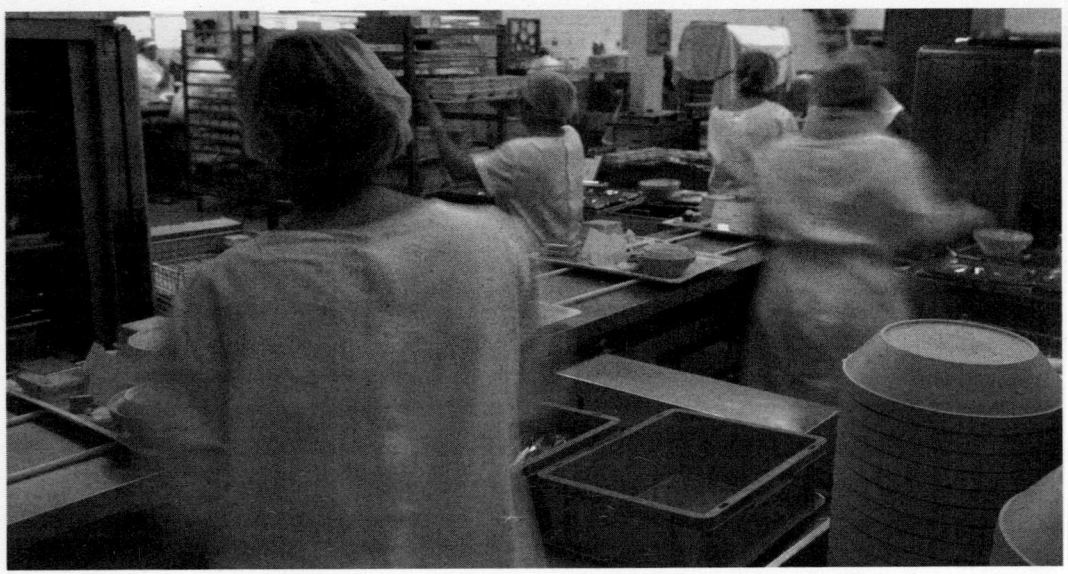

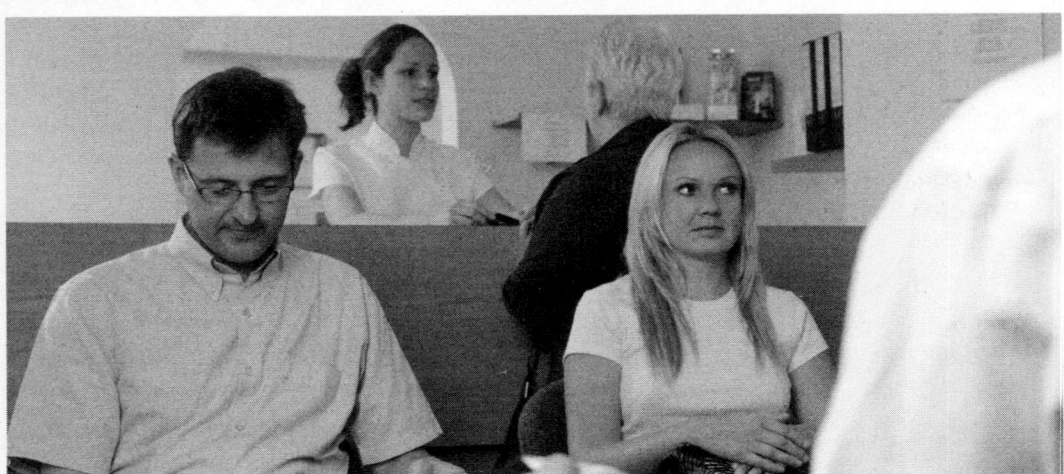

Photo 1.2 A profession is much wider than people may at first think, and being interprofessional includes working with all the people you come into contact with and who have an effect on patients or clients, such as caterers and reception staff. Dr Heinz Linke/iStock; Catherine Yeulet/iStock.

of people who have undertaken a given programme of education and/or training, and as a result of this are permitted to become part of a much larger and somewhat exclusive group. Traditionally, the professions were law, medicine and the Church; many others, relevant to services discussed in this book, are now recognized by law in the UK and other countries – for example, social work, teaching, physiotherapy, radiography, speech and language therapy. In Box 1.3 you will find a very brief outline of some of the

---

Box 1.3: What is a professional? Information and further reading

A **profession** acts collectively to restrict access to rewards (e.g., remuneration or social status) through establishing criteria by which others, non-members, are excluded. They lay claim to specialist knowledge and this underpins the services they offer; they exercise control of their knowledge and thus autonomy over their area of work. Each profession has a unique culture, influenced by its own values and beliefs. Through the education and training practices of a profession, its members are socialized into the professional culture and, in this way, practitioners from a particular profession adopt certain attitudes and conduct their practice in certain ways. In the UK a profession has the right to self-regulation; other countries construe professionals differently; so, for example, in continental Europe they are seen as 'elite administrators possessing their offices by virtue of academic credentials' (Collins 1990). A **member of a profession** can use a title, e.g., occupational therapist, and this title is restricted by law to them.

Further reading on the professions and professionalism

Freidson E. (1994) *Professionalism Reborn: Theory, Prophecy and Policy.* Cambridge: Polity.
Freidson, E. (2001) *Professionalism: The Third Logic.* Cambridge: Polity.
Leicht, K. T. and Fennell, M. L. (2001) *Professional Work: A Sociological Approach.* Oxford: Blackwell.
Macdonald, K. M. (1995) *The Sociology of the Professions.* London: Sage.

---

characteristics that define a profession and a list of further reading on this topic. The books recommended discuss general theoretical aspects of professionalism in some depth: for specialist writing in respect of any one profession, we suggest you search an appropriate database such as ASSIA, CINAHL, PSYCHINFO, SCIE, ERIC or Medline.

As the information in Box 1.3 indicates, a programme of professional education or training aims to equip its learners with the required knowledge and skills, and to socialize them into the culture of that profession. In this way, new social work graduates work with the values and beliefs expected of a social worker; school teachers conduct themselves with the attitudes expected of the teaching profession; similarly, nursing/medical students learn how to be nurses/doctors, and the same applies to all other health and social care workers.

For today's students, the process of professional socialization is undertaken alongside learning to become part of the interprofessional community of practitioners. This can be difficult and can lead to the assumption that professional values and beliefs are the same as interprofessional values and beliefs. We think there are some key differences between being professional and being interprofessional, but looking at how to be professional can help us to see how to be interprofessional. Our model of being interprofessional shows that this is really all about what happens at the boundary between one person and another, and about how good the relationships across this boundary are. Meads and Ashcroft (2005) set out a useful framework for who might need to form relationships in interprofessional working teams, for example, policy-makers, service users, practitioners from other professions and working groups, and the public. We would add carers of service users to this list, and remind you that all or any of these people may be involved in a given collaborative working situation.

With this in mind, we have started a list of professional ways of practising as an interprofessional worker. One of these is about being respectful of everyone in the collaborative team. This includes the user of services and could include people such as advocates, who you may be meeting for the first time and who you know very little about. They might have different ethical, professional and philosophical frameworks. Part of being interprofessional is learning to acknowledge different professional frameworks and being prepared to negotiate across the boundaries. Doctors, for example, have traditionally seen themselves less as part of the team and more as leaders of all their other colleagues: this relates to many of the aspects of their profession that we highlighted in Box 1.2. Social workers have a strong tradition of anti-oppressive practice that highlights oppression due to race, gender, sexuality, disability, class, age and ethnicity. Learning to work with colleagues with different frameworks is part of being interprofessional.

When people with different life experiences, different levels of expertise and in different roles work together, there is the potential for the power that experiences and expertise confer to interfere with the need to be respectful. Learner Exercise 1.3 is designed to help you understand how the power that people think they have might have an impact in an interprofessional team. You can either use the examples we've given (a disabled child and an occupational therapist) or similar people from your own work setting. If you work in a school, the pair might be a head teacher and a parent. For each person, make some notes about their experiences and expertise: how much they have, where this comes from and how valuable it is. We've put in two already to give you a start and we've also rated how much power these give, using a star system. There are no right or wrong answers to this: the point is to think about the overall power rating of each person and how this might affect their ability to have respect for the opinions and ideas of the other person.

Another aspect of how to be interprofessional concerns recognizing that while collaborative working is primarily about making sure we deliver the best service possible to our clients,

Learner Exercise 1.3: Respect and power in the interprofessional team

	Disabled child	Occupational therapist
Expertise		Professional qualifications
Experience	Lifetime of being a wheelchair user	
Overall power	***	****

there is, arguably, an equal imperative to care for each other in the workplace. Recognizing yourself as a team member involves widening your horizons to include not only a duty of care to users of services, but also a duty of care to each other. The simple principle that

> . . . my working and professional practices should not harm me, or permit me to harm others who work with me . . .

offers a way of assessing how we conduct ourselves. It is part of our professional attitude to being interprofessional.

Also on our list of ways to be interprofessional is the need to value both your own knowledge and what others know. This includes knowing when it is in the service user's best interest for you to share your knowledge with someone else. An example of this is the wisdom of the physiotherapist who teaches nursing colleagues how to deliver some basic physiotherapy to someone who has had a stroke. There is often only one physiotherapist for many patients, and the physiotherapist is likely to be responsible for patients on more than one hospital ward. Having an open attitude which allows the nurses in regular contact with the patient to deliver therapy that will aid their recovery is clearly working in an interprofessional way for patient benefit. Similarly, speech and language therapists teach parents the basic skills necessary for their child to have daily therapy for a speech impediment: respecting their role in the joint care of their child. In both these examples being interprofessional means initiating an explicit ripple outwards, from one to many, of knowledge and skills in order to better meet the service users' needs.

Our list of how to act interprofessionally is summarized in Box 1.4. We suggest that these are core values that support a culture of being interprofessional. It is not an exhaustive list (you may be able to add to it), but someone working in this way is working interprofessionally and, as you can see in Figure 1.4, we have added this third vital dimension into our final model of what being interprofessional means. In Box 1.5 what you need to know, the skills needed to apply this knowledge and the attitudes that mean

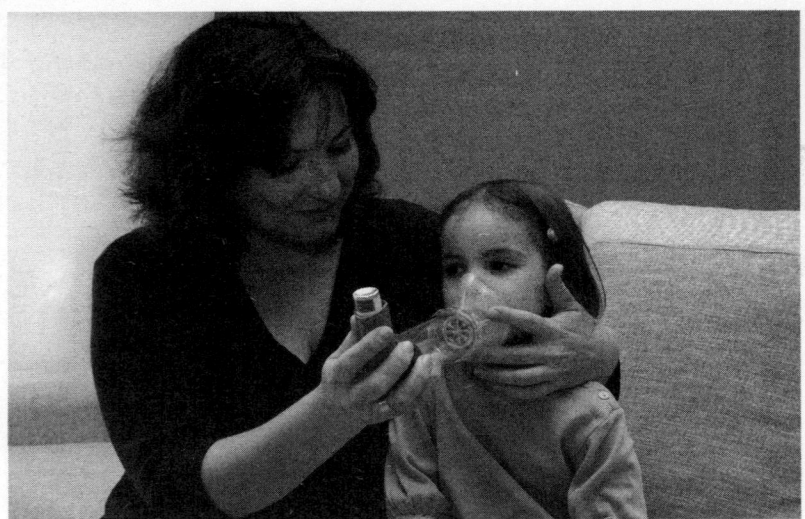

Photo 1.3 Being interprofessional can mean initiating a ripple of knowledge outwards, from specialists to service users or their friends and family. Xavier Gallego/iStock.

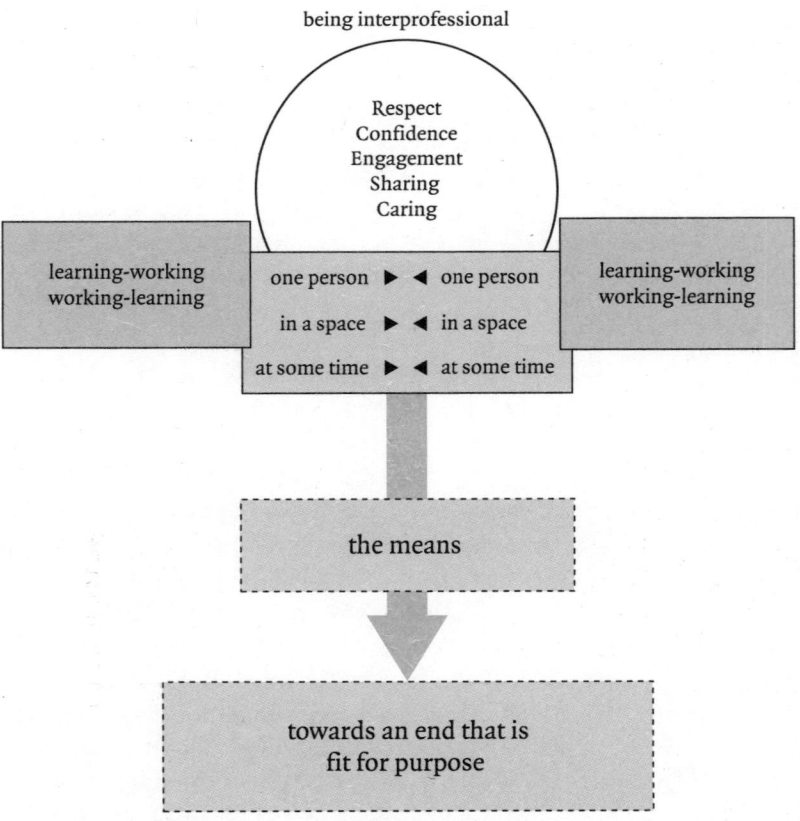

Figure 1.4 Our final model of being interprofessional

Box 1.4: Core values of being interprofessional include having:

Respect for everyone in the collaborative team.
Confidence in what you know and what you don't know, and in what others know.
A willingness to engage with others rather than taking a detached view of proceedings.
A caring disposition towards your colleagues.
An approachable attitude and showing a willingness to share what you know as a means to the best possible outcome for the user of your service.

Box 1.5: Summary of first-post competencies for being an interprofessional practitioner

Knowledge

Understand the role and working context of other practitioners and begin to identify how these interrelate.
Recognize the range of knowledge and skills of all other colleagues.
Understand the principles and practice of effective teamwork.

Skills

Apply sound verbal and written communication methods with colleagues from other work settings.
Identify situations where collaboration is helpful or essential.
Work collaboratively with service users and carers.
Use interprofessional learning in work settings.

Attitudes

Appreciate the value of interprofessional collaboration.
Acknowledge and respect others' views, values and ideas.

this is done in the right way are set out. Combining the knowledge, skills and attitudes in Box 1.5 in a mindful way enables you to be a competent interprofessional practitioner. Note that these are basic competencies, expected of a practitioner in their first post. As your career develops and you attain more senior positions, your role may require you to have more advanced interprofessional competencies. We write about these in the last chapter of the book. What remains the same are the values (Box 1.4) that underpin all these competencies.

To conclude

In this chapter we identified what being interprofessional is and what knowledge, skills and attitudes are needed to practise in this way. We considered some areas in which interprofessional practice might take place and illustrated some of their complexities. In the next chapter we introduce you to some historical and current imperatives for collaborative care, including client-focused services and professional fulfilment. We look at why learning and working together, as part of interprofessional practice, are suggested as solutions to some of the failures in service delivery and at some key principles of working interprofessionally.

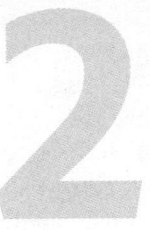

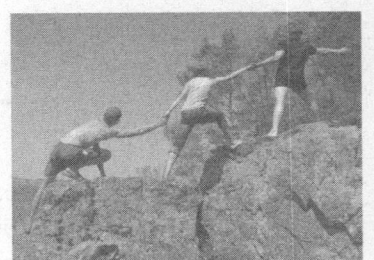

Being Interprofessional: Imperatives and Key Principles

With the possible exception of the equator, everything begins somewhere.

C. S. Lewis

What you will read in this chapter

We hope you now have a picture of what being interprofessional is and the knowledge, skills and attitudes needed to practise in this way. Now we want to turn to why the ability to be interprofessional is an essential part of being a professional worker. We summarize some of the historical and current imperatives behind the movements for being interprofessional and working collaboratively with others. Then we introduce some key principles of interprofessional working.

The past and being interprofessional

The busy nature of the model of being interprofessional in chapter 1 (Figure 1.4), signals that this is not a simple way of working. As we discussed in chapter 1, different public service professions came into being in different ways; they have their own histories, professional cultures, ethical and value bases, training and career trajectories. Being interprofessional is partly about learning to understand and work with the professional values and cultures of others.

An interprofessional approach to delivering health services contrasts strongly with the traditional ways of working in health care. These can be characterized as being led by certain long-standing, high-status, and some would say privileged, professional groups. Freidson (1970a, b) explains that medicine has long been the dominant professional group, with doctors holding positions of authority. This can create challenges within an interprofessional team. Education and practice within health care has also been dominated by the hospital setting, although that is changing along with the greater emphasis now being on primary care. In contrast, social work is often delivered in a community setting. It has a diverse history and came into being through a mixture of the Poor Law, charitable works, religious foundations and radical reformers. These influences are reflected in a professional culture which is concerned with social integration, social justice and strengthening social functioning.

To deliver modern-day services to some client groups, it is important that health and social agencies work closely together: yet they might have different frameworks and priorities. Being interprofessional is about being able to acknowledge and negotiate these kinds of differences.

Values and ethics and being interprofessional

Service user and carer involvement emerge as common themes in many codes of professional practice. There are, however, similarities and differences in the professional values and ethical frameworks that practitioners in different professions work to (Box 2.1). For example, the nursing code of professional conduct refers to a client's uniqueness and dignity, whereby care is to be provided irrespective of a patient's ethnicity, religious beliefs and/or personal attributes. The code of ethics for social workers refers to 'group' as well as individual differences; thereby locating people in their collective, social and cultural context and bringing in a notion of 'structural inequalities', e.g., the disadvantage associated with elements such as class, race and gender (Wilmott 1995). This can affect working practices and service delivery, as well as interprofessional learning and working. Learner Exercise 2.1 is designed so that you can reflect on some of the different professional codes of conduct, and consider how they might inform and impact on interprofessional practice.

Box 2.1: A comparison of two codes of professional conduct

Wilmott (1995), comparing the UKCC statutory Code of Professional Conduct for nurses with the 1986 British Association of Social Workers (BASW) Code of Ethics of Social Workers (later updated to the GSCC Codes of Practice 2002), found that:

> Whilst the UKCC required nurses to serve the interest of society and justify public confidence, the BASW code gave a more active dimension to the social worker's role in terms of social policy planning and action. A legitimate area for action by social workers is to critique society and its structures. Therefore, the relationship between the state and society is an area for action by social workers but not by nurses as such, and thus reveals the political dimension to the social worker's responsibility.

Learner Exercise 2.1: Different codes of practice and learning and working interprofessionally

First, consult the code of ethics of your professional association and the codes of ethics of two other professional groups. Consider their similarities and differences and write these down as lists or brief statements. We suggest that you lay them out as three columns.

Looking across all three columns, highlight in one colour the general statements of principle and, in another colour, the more practical guidance or rules. Looking at the results of this, are there distinctions related to topics or professions? You might also like to attempt to explain any differences by using your own profession as the starting point.

Again, considering your three columns, how do you feel the following areas are represented?

- Promoting individual service users' rights
- Promoting effective practice
- Protecting service users and the public
- Challenging inequality
- Promoting social justice.

Are there any references to qualities of character, e.g., honesty?
    Finally, consider:

1. How useful are these codes in protecting service users and in guiding practitioners?

And:

2. What are their implications for interprofessional working across professions?

(Adapted from Banks 2006)

Other influences on being interprofessional

Barriers to interprofessional learning, and thus to being interprofessional in practice, also arise from the tradition of separate education and training for different professional groups. The medical dominance noted earlier has been reflected in the history of professional education within the health-care sciences, including nursing and the allied health professions. These are now independent, but for many years the medical profession exercised control over their curricula, examinations and professional registration. Learning together as teachers, police, social workers and health practitioners is still relatively new. Where education takes place also affects interprofessional working. For example, hospital settings and primary health-care practices are key places in the practice-based education of most health-care practitioners, while social workers undertake their practice learning largely in the community and teachers do this in schools.

So, given this history, what were the influences that led practitioners away from well-rooted customs to adopt different behaviours that would enable services to be delivered in new and potentially complex ways? What were the key pressure points for changes in initial and continuing education and training programmes that, in many places, led to the introduction of at least some interprofessional education, either on the campus or in service settings?

For a detailed overview of the major international and regional (European, North American, Australasian and Developing Countries) reports and developments calling for interprofessional education and practice, we suggest you read Meads and Barr (2005). One of the most important early reports came from the World Health Organisation (WHO) and they have recently confirmed this (Box 2.2).

Box 2.2: Views of the World Health Organisation on interprofessional education and collaborative practice

The report of the World Health Organisation's 1987 Study Group on Multiprofessional Education for Health Personnel, *Learning Together to Work Together for Health*, is considered to be one of the most significant and authoritative calls for interprofessional education and collaborative practice, inspiring movements to improve health outcomes globally, such as community-based health and social care services (World Health Organisation 1987).

In 2008, the WHO reaffirmed its interest in interprofessional education and collaborative practice as a means of improving global health outcomes, with the planned publication of *Framework for Action on Interprofessional Education & Collaborative Practice*, asserting that:

> The World Health Organisation recognizes interprofessional collaboration in education and practice as an innovative strategy that will play an important role in mitigating the global health workforce crisis (and) interprofessional education is a necessary step in preparing a 'collaborative practice-ready' health workforce. (World Health Organisation forthcoming)

You might well question the relevance of knowing how it was in the past. You might argue that these calls have a long pedigree, as the quote from Gillies et al. (2004) below shows. Surely things have changed, or at least it is all in the process of changing? In some places, yes; others, to some extent; and, some would say, for many services little has changed yet. We believe that some understanding of the history of interprofessional education and practice can reinforce its importance for today's students. During your experience in the workplace you are likely to have seen that there is clearly more to do yet. Your learning about being interprofessional will help this to happen.

> The imperative for effective collaborative practice across and between professions has existed in policy papers for decades and has accelerated significantly and in sharper definition in the last 5 years. (Gillies et al. 2004)

To continue with our focus on some of the major imperatives for collaborative working in the United Kingdom, we offer three ways of looking at these (adapted from Meads and Ashcroft, 2005):

1. Good practice guidelines that address identified health needs and contain lessons from past errors to act as crisis prevention tools.
2. Performance-shaped changes in reconfigured statuary sectors, often working with the community and voluntary and private sectors.
3. Personal and organizational development-driven changes in practice, which in turn impact on service users and their carers.

Good practice guidelines and crisis prevention

Many agencies (local and national), professional bodies and other organizations produce guidelines and improvement action plans targeted at the care of specific groups of patients. Very often these have arisen from identifying the need for improved heath and well-being outcomes. The National Clinical Guidelines for Stroke detailed below are one example where an interprofessional approach is recommended. One of their recommendations is as follows.

A specialist stroke team should include staff with specialist knowledge of stroke, specifically:

  i) a consultant physician specialising in stroke medicine
 ii) nurses
iii) a physiotherapist
 iv) an occupational therapist
  v) a speech and language therapist
 vi) a neuroradiologist
vii) a dietitian
viii) a clinical psychologist
 ix) a pharmacist
  x) a social worker.

(Intercollegiate Stroke Working Party 2004, p. 16; a third edition of these guidelines is now available)

Another example comes from Walsall, where service providers recognized the need to improve health outcomes in maternity care. They commissioned a study into risk factors in relation to low birth weight babies, which recommended several actions under the heading of inter-agency and interprofessional working:

- Establish joint inter-agency posts for low birth weight prevention targeting the most vulnerable and marginalised groups of society.
- Implement a common assessment tool for all pregnant girls and women.
- Establish inter-agency forum for low birth weight reduction.
- Promote multi-agency strategies in the provision of preconception advice.
- Agree lead agency and key workers for complex cases.
- Adopt a more integrated model for all services.
- Ensure effective networking to improve services across all care sectors.
- Raise the profile of Patient and Public Involvement thus 'giving people what they want'.
- Implement earlier proactive interventions, before pregnancy and raising awareness of low birth weight.
- Consider future developments through pooled budgets. (Tope et al. 2008, p. 11)

In relation to crisis prevention, two reports (in 2001 and 2003) highlighted that much more attention needed to be paid to the ways in which practitioners from different professions worked together. The report of Lord Laming on the findings of the inquiry into the death of Victoria Climbié (Laming 2003) and that of Sir Ian Kennedy on the inquiry into paediatric open-heart surgery at the Bristol Royal Infirmary (Kennedy et al. 2001) are constantly cited as reasons why practitioners should be interprofessional. Both provide more than sufficient evidence for the importance of collaborative working and the imperative for this to be part of the professional role of all those who work in health and social care settings. Both had significant things to say about the nature of being interprofessional, as shown by the examples in the quotes below.

Teamwork is the collaborative effort of all. . .patients do not belong to any one profession: they are the responsibility of all who take care of them.

(Kennedy et al. 2001, p. 277)

. . . need. . .to document information. . .to share that information and to ensure subsequently that what has been agreed is carried through. (Laming 2003, p. 283)

Performance related

Performance-related drivers for interprofessional working arise from changes in the nature of twenty-first-century public services. These are now much more target driven, require greater accountability of budgets and the demonstration of governance systems for patient/ client safety. The 1980s saw the introduction of the idea that the client of public services should be regarded as an active customer with choices rather than as a grateful recipient. In some areas this has led to service users having more say about how services are delivered to them. This idea was taken from the private sector and the market economy and has underpinned the marketization of public services. This (and other changes) led to practice reforms and updated management models.

Originally, and typically, management models for health services were based on military systems, systems that were mirrored in many industrial or workplace practices. Generally, this can be understood as a top-down/hierarchical model, within which the subordinate levels are given – and expected to carry out – orders. These processes also linked to the class system and to the dominance of practitioners from high-status professions, as we discussed earlier. Social work and education services were delivered in diverse ways, depending on their setting. Services in the voluntary sector have traditionally been delivered in a more informal and flexible way than those in the statutory sector, although there is pressure to bring in similar management systems here as well.

Nowadays, the complexity of managing and delivering public services such as health care, social care and education means that

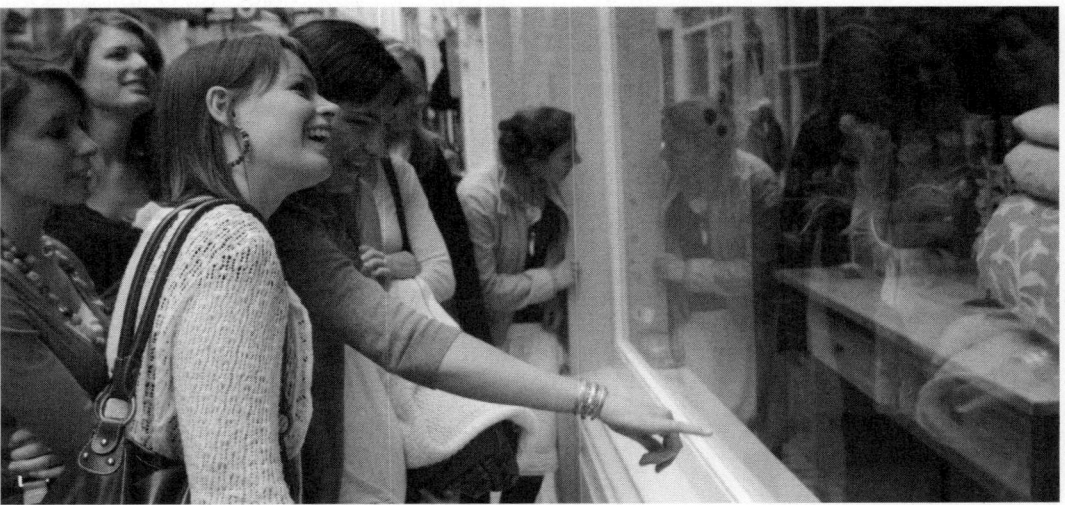

Photo 2.1 The marketization of public services means that clients and patients are more like customers who have a choice what services they use, and how they use them. Paul Piebinga/iStock.

the knowledge, the skills and service delivery cannot be collected in a meaningful way around a single role or a single person. Interprofessional working is becoming the mechanism through which diverse talents are harnessed to deliver effective and efficient services. In practice, this is a model that acts as a rotating wheel, with the *most appropriate* person or human services agency leading at any given stage during the service user's journey. Leading the interprofessional team becomes contingent upon the specific needs of the service user. You will read much more about user-focused services in Part II of this book.

Development related

Being interprofessional as part of professional practice is often related to the way a service develops in its local context. National developments also play a part in organizational and service changes. The professional and personal development of people is also important; helping to change what needs to change. In this way, externally driven changes influence the lives of service users and those working to deliver services. We briefly look at some examples of these drives towards interprofessional working next.

For service development, one of the clearest examples is the comparison between current health care and what could actually be offered to patients when the UK National Health Service began in 1946. With advances in science and technology in all fields, care has become more complex. With complexity comes the need to draw on the different sets of knowledge and skills: what is known about a particular field of work is distributed amongst several practitioners. For effective and safe delivery of services the work has to be arranged so that the distributed knowledge is harnessed. The interprofessional service delivery wheel has distributed knowledge circulating around it. An example of this is the inclusive membership of the group responsible for writing the National Clinical Guidelines for Stroke, referred to above. Amongst the members were a dietician, economist, occupational therapist, pharmacist, physician, psychologist, speech and language therapist, a member of the Stroke Association: different people contributing their collective and unique knowledge. The result is a set of valuable working guidelines for all practitioners working together towards more effective care of patients who have had a stroke.

New challenges to our health and social well-being present themselves all the time. This is often followed by the requirement for changes in the way services are offered. In response, organizations are reconfigured and practitioner roles and ways of working change. Youth Crime Teams described by Anning et al. (2006) arose from the 1998 Crime and Disorder Act. This meant that, by law, teams dealing with offending by children and young people had to include at least:

- One social worker
- One probation officer
- One police officer
- Someone from the local health authority
- The local chief education officer.

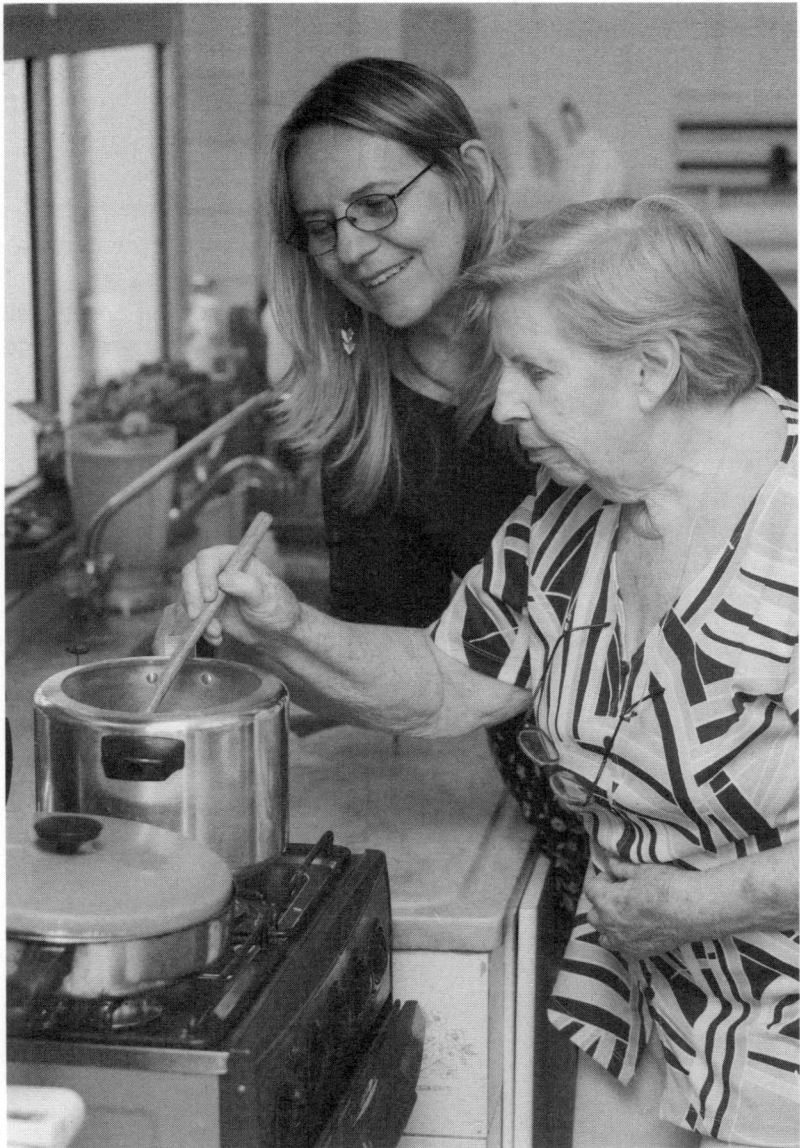

Photo 2.2 A patient recovering from a stroke will need the help of many professionals, long after they suffer the stroke. For example, occupational therapists will assess whether the patient can continue to perform the roles they did before the stroke; it is important for all professionals to understand one another and not work in opposition either knowingly or unknowingly. Orangelinemedia/iStock.

In Anning et al. (2006) you can read more about this team which worked together in one place, was funded by many different agencies and had staff from many services working interprofessionaly. Note that a 1996 report into youth offending had noted that there was:

> . . . a lack of joined-up thinking. . .inefficient deployment of resources. . .delays in processing youth offenders in the criminal justice system. (p. 32)

Finally, as the quote from Gillies et al. below highlights, interprofessional practice is beneficial for those delivering and receiving services. One example of this is the way people with learning disabilities work with staff from diverse professional backgrounds to enable people with learning disabilities to lead fulfilling lives. A website search will produce many examples of this. On <http://www.learningdisabilities.org.uk> we found a jointly written booklet that can help these young people lead full and fulfilling lives. The organization behind this is called Generate. In Box 2.3 we've put some details about this but you can find out a lot more by going to this website.

The benefits of effective inter-professional practice are identified as including the sharing of knowledge and resources, enabling a more satisfying and supportive work environment, the widening of professional perspectives,

---

Box 2.3: Details of a publication written with service users

All about feeling down

A booklet for young people with learning disabilities
Words by Ruth Townsley and Julian Goodwin,
Norah Fry Research Centre, University of Bristol

Thank you to the young people and staff at Warmley Park School in Bristol and Emma Wilson, Charlotte Hall and Nick McKerrow from Generate for their help with making this booklet. They looked at the words and pictures and said what they thought. We listened to their ideas, then changed things to make the booklet better.

About this booklet
This booklet is for young people with learning disabilities aged 14 to 25. This booklet is about what you can do if you feel down. It would be a good idea to ask someone you trust to help you think and talk about things in the booklet. You might want to ask them to read it with you. As you grow up, changes can feel hard to deal with. But there can be exciting times too. Everyone has ups and downs, especially about growing up.

encouraging overall service planning, achieving objectives
more fully and economically and maximising specialist skills
with resulting positive outcomes for service users.

(Gillies et al. 2004, p. 3)

Changing practices

Working interprofessionaly can mean that practitioners have
opportunities for professional development through collaborative
working that focuses on who is best placed to provide optimal
service delivery for users. In cancer care, collaborative initiatives have
reshaped working practices to introduce radiographer-led treatment
review and radiographer-prescribing for the management of treatment
toxicity (Francis and Hogg 2006). These roles mean improved patient
care and give development opportunities for practitioners. For these
changes to take place, radiography, medical and pharmacy colleagues
needed to learn about, from and with each other.

These and similar interprofessional collaborations can give rise to
mixed feelings about aspects of identity and boundaries. It is worth
remembering that sometimes to gain something we may have to give
something up.

Key principles for interprofessional working

We have emphasized the complexity of working interprofessionally
in this chapter, and following chapters demonstrate this in many
different ways. So it's unsurprising that the staff involved experience
both highs and lows in roles that ask them to be interprofessional.
The very experience of recognizing when something positive arises
from collaborating with others, as well as the not-so-good aspects,
contributes to our professional development.

To be a professional, effective and interprofessional practitioner
it's important to recognize that interprofessional working is
not simply a response to protocols or guidelines, but rather the
adoption of principles and values. Essentially, this is a shift away
from directives about what anyone must and should do towards
encouraging the attitudes that foster interprofessional and user-
focused collaboration.

In Box 2.4 we set out some key principles about working
interprofessionally. These principles are underpinned by values, and
our hope is that they will serve as markers along your route to being
interprofessional.

With the key principles in Box 2.4 in mind, take a moment to
look at Pause Point 2.1. Its aim is to help you think through how this
applies to you. We include some starters to show different aspects for
staff of being interprofessional: these are all quotes by practitioners
given to researchers. The rest of the space is blank for you to fill

Box 2.4: Key principles of being interprofessional

1. The willingness and capability to work both collaboratively and inclusively.
2. An understanding of the nature and extent of your duty of care both to those who use your services and to your colleagues.
3. Ensuring that your interprofessional work is underpinned with the following attitudes towards everyone you work with and for: respect, confidence, engagement, willingness to negotiate and readiness to share.
4. The willingness and capability to communicate clearly what you want and believe; and to listen to what others want and believe.
5. The commitment and capability to develop and deliver mutually acceptable shared plans.
6. The willingness and capability to contribute to shaping change and to welcome contributions from a spectrum of other stakeholders in the services you offer.

Pause Point 2.1: Being interprofessional

- 'It's made me think about what I don't do and what I can't do as much as what I can do' (Anning et al. 2006, p. 74)
- 'It's not about saying I'm a social worker and I can only do this and I'm a nurse and I can only do this, because that's what service users tell us they don't want' (Taylor et al. 2006, p. 102)
- 'I do feel a lack of clarity about my professional role' (Anning et al. 2006, p. 73)
- 'It's broken down a few barriers working with the paediatricians' (Anning et al. 2006, p. 74)

Now add your thoughts on being interprofessional . . .

in. Have a go now and then return to it later on, perhaps after you have been out on a placement where interprofessional working is happening, or when you've read other chapters in this book.

To conclude

In 2008 the WHO reminded us that:

> In the 21st century, health is a shared responsibility, involving equitable access to essential care and collective defence against transnational threats. (<www.who.int>; accessed 3 January 2008)

The calls for collaboration reviewed here suggest that this imperative does not apply only to health. All human services and the people who work in them need to share responsibility for delivery, with each other, with service users and with unpaid carers. All these people need to work together interprofessionally.

In 2005 our colleagues Geoff Meads and John Ashcroft said:

Being professional today means becoming interprofessional.

We have argued in this chapter that optimal service delivery depends on practitioners who have the knowledge, skills and attitudes that enable them to be interprofessional. Both now and in the future, being professional includes being interprofessional.

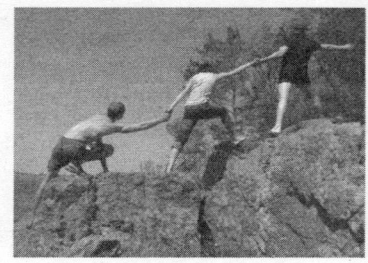

3

Learning and Working in Teams

Let there be spaces in your togetherness.

Kahlil Gibran

What you will read in this chapter

Being interprofessional, as a way of promoting effective service delivery, means learning and working in a variety of teams. In this chapter we explore aspects of being an effective team member; and how you might understand more fully people's actions and activities within the team.

Teams and team-working have a long history in many fields of work and play: many sports and hobbies depend on team participation. Likewise, the delivery of community services, for example, probation services and care of older people, has always relied on staff from more than one specialism. Teams of practitioners work together for many reasons. For instance, the complexity of giving radiotherapy means that radiographers work in teams of two to three. Where twenty-four-hour care is needed several staff form a team with rotating membership, which ensures that round-the-clock cover is provided.

Most people who use public and private services come into contact with practitioners from more than one service and more than one profession. It is important that practitioners communicate effectively and work as a collaborative interprofessional, and often inter-agency, team. In this way you put *being interprofessional*, as we described this way of being in chapter 1, into your working practice. This is easily stated and obviously reasonable, but not always easy to achieve, as the scenario about Lena, a community worker, and Gemma, in chapter 9 (p. 176) shows.

We believe that many of the studies of the way teams succeed at the art of collaboration can be helpful for learning more about being interprofessional in a team. This chapter discusses some key aspects:

- Elements of effective team-working
- Being a member of a team
- Behaviour and emotions in the team
- The life cycle of a team
- Leadership in interprofessional teams
- Team members as team types; and
- Types and purposes of teams.

Effective team-working

Team work sits at the centre of all interprofessional working and collaboration, and the input of each team member is integral to creating the team's practice. Every person's way of being with others in the team forms the connections that are the *make-or-break* elements of team-working. We have all heard the phrase 'a chain is as strong as its weakest link' – and this sentiment readily fits interprofessional and other team-working contexts. Some key characteristics of a team – what it is, what makes a team work well and how teams become successful – are shown in the quotes below. These quotes come from work by researchers interested in the performance of business teams (Katzenbach and Smith 1993, p. 9). We've used their work because we believe that all teams who work together over a period of time have things in common: good teams that work well share characteristics with each other. We can learn from how teams in other professions work: an example of interprofessional learning.

> a small number of people with complimentary skills, who are committed to a common purpose, performance, goals and approach, for which they are mutually accountable . . .
>
> Real teams are deeply committed to their purpose, goals and approach . . .
>
> High performance team members are. . .committed to one another

Many teams in community services and health care come together around a specific task, which might have a very short duration, particularly in emergency care. The team is formed from the people with the right skills who are available at the time. When their immediate work is complete they disband and they are unlikely to meet on future occasions as exactly the same team. In these circumstances the insights into team-working that are based on longevity and phases of development will be less applicable. The most important need will be for the individuals present to have honed their team-work skills so that they can work productively within a wide range of *teams of the moment*. This

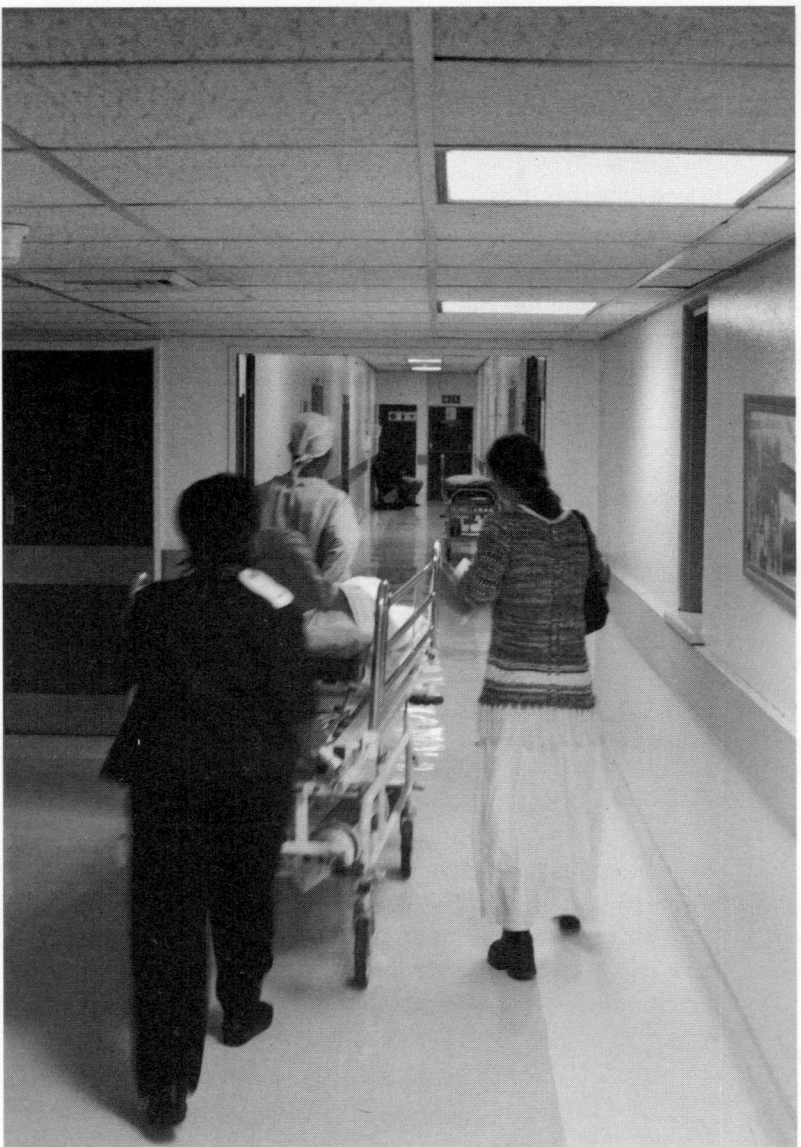

Photo 3.1 In an emergency, a team will come together quickly – for example, various medical staff and an interpreter if the patient cannot speak English; the members may not have met before and may not work together again, but they need to be able to cooperate effectively in the emergency. Poco_bw/iStock.

skill development proceeds by developing an understanding of principles that apply to most teams, coming to know the characteristics of the types of teams which your area of practice uses and making a conscious effort to think about the group dynamics you encounter (see Learner Exercise 3.1) . It involves knowing the quality of your own contributions and what you can learn from the quality of others' contributions.

Learner Exercise 3.1: Your teams and their characteristics

List five or six teams of which you have experience. Make them as diverse as
possible. These may be workplace teams or teams drawn from other aspects of
your life.

To what extent do the phrases quoted in the boxes above resonate with the teams
you have listed?

Which teams had a reasonably stable membership, working together over a period
of weeks, months or even years? Which were transitory *teams of the moment*?

In what ways did working with each of these teams feel different, raise different
challenges and provide different rewards?

Box 3.1: Positive ways to behave during team work

Share relevant practice knowledge so that others know <u>from</u> you <u>about</u> aspects of
importance to the service user or way of delivering a service.

Agree practice and/or management processes for service users and the team.

Understand the values, knowledge and skills of others in the team – so that the
team's working practices can harmonise and use everyone's contribution (where
appropriate).

Work towards creating effective ways of working together – for example, agreeing
ground-rules for the team.

Actively participate as team members.

Listen to and engage in discussions, including problem-solving, with the team.

Take responsibility to communicate effectively with and beyond the team.

Strive to maintain a professional relationship with team members and others
affected by the team.

Engage in the team assessment of processes. For example; what to start doing,
continue doing and/or stop doing – and the actions needed to meet team goals.

Management and business perspectives say that when you are part
of a team you are expected to work to the agreed goals or purpose
of the team and to share values such as a commitment to the team's
goals and to each other. These commonalities are the glue that holds
the team together. This doesn't mean that everyone in the team
will always agree. It does mean that raising and resolving problems
should fit agreed patterns of behaviour. Box 3.1 contains a set of
positive ways of working in teams, including interprofessional teams.
If all teams functioned using these ideas and ideals, then service
delivery would be much more effective and the users of services would
feel more satisfied with what happens.

Note how many of the expectations in Box 3.1 are similar to most
of the key features of being interprofessional that you read about in
chapter 1. In the same way as we wrote about being interprofessional
as an active state, team-working means actively engaging with

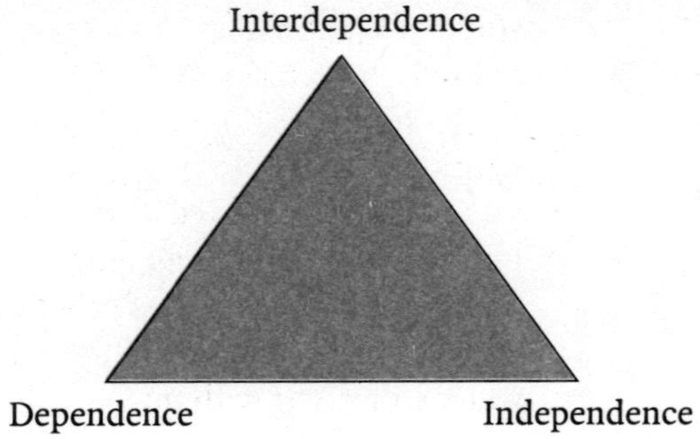

Interdependence

Dependence   Independence

Figure 3.1 Balanced dependency as a way of being in a team

the team's goals and purposes so that these are understood and
embraced by all team members. To do this you have to know when
to be assertive, when to reshape your ideas around those of others
and when to learn from others. One way of looking at this way of
behaving is by recognizing the importance of all members of the
team:

- Recognizing their need to depend on others
- Being able to blend with others; and
- Having confidence in yourself and others.

Figure 3.1 demonstrates the balanced interplay between these
different ways of being dependent in a team: independent; dependent
on others; interdependent with others.

   As an individual practitioner, being in any team and being
interprofessional means learning to manage your role with each of
these three elements in mind. In later chapters we discuss how new
service configurations and contemporary practice depend on staff
being able to recognize where they should be in the model in Figure
3.1, for each and every aspect of their practice.

Being a member of a team

From what you have read so far, you've probably realized that what
a team is and how successful it is depends almost entirely on the
members of that team. So we now look at being a member of a team,
and specifically relate this to being interprofessional in a team. Our
aim is to highlight some ways of participating that help you to feel
good about being in a team and some hints about the sort of team
person you are.

   A major issue for service delivery teams relates to how people
normally behave at work. We probably all know from experience that
being part of a team is not always straightforward. Some of you may
have watched colleagues struggle to participate in a particular team;
seen someone who perhaps should know better become a problem
to the rest of the team. It's easy for this to happen, but if we know

some of the things that make or break the work of a team this can be helpful.

To start with, successful team-working depends on how willing we are to commit to being a team member. In the opening sections of this chapter we looked at some rather broad attributes of team work, like sharing values and being committed to the team. Learner Exercise 3.2 aims to help you think about these aspects in relation to you as part of a team. It asks you to focus on the team-work environments you are involved with now or have previously worked in. We suggest you write your answers to questions 1 to 9 in the box, then look at question 10 to reflect more deeply on your understanding of the context that you are working in. If you have time repeat the exercise for another team: after all, we behave differently in different teams. If you can't think of a work team, do the exercise using a sports team, or a voluntary group you work with.

Learner Exercise 3.2: Me and my teams

Questions about a team you work in/have worked in	Your answers

1. What is the purpose and function of the team?
2. Who makes up the team?
3. Does the team have an agreed process and/or a pattern of work, or does it appear to function in an ad hoc way?
4. Is everyone in the team equal? What is the purpose and effect of any inequality?
5. Are the team roles equal? What is the purpose and effect of any inequality?
6. What is the decision-making process in the team? Does this process work well for all contributors?
7. Are any work settings in the team represented by more than one person? How does this affect the dynamics of communication and decision-making?
8. Does the team interact outside the task environment?
9. In your view, do the team members 'know' each other?

Question 10	Your answers
Look at your answers; can you see any patterns emerging that relate to how you feel about your commitment to that team? What do your answers tell you about how effective teams are made, and how they operate and manage themselves?	

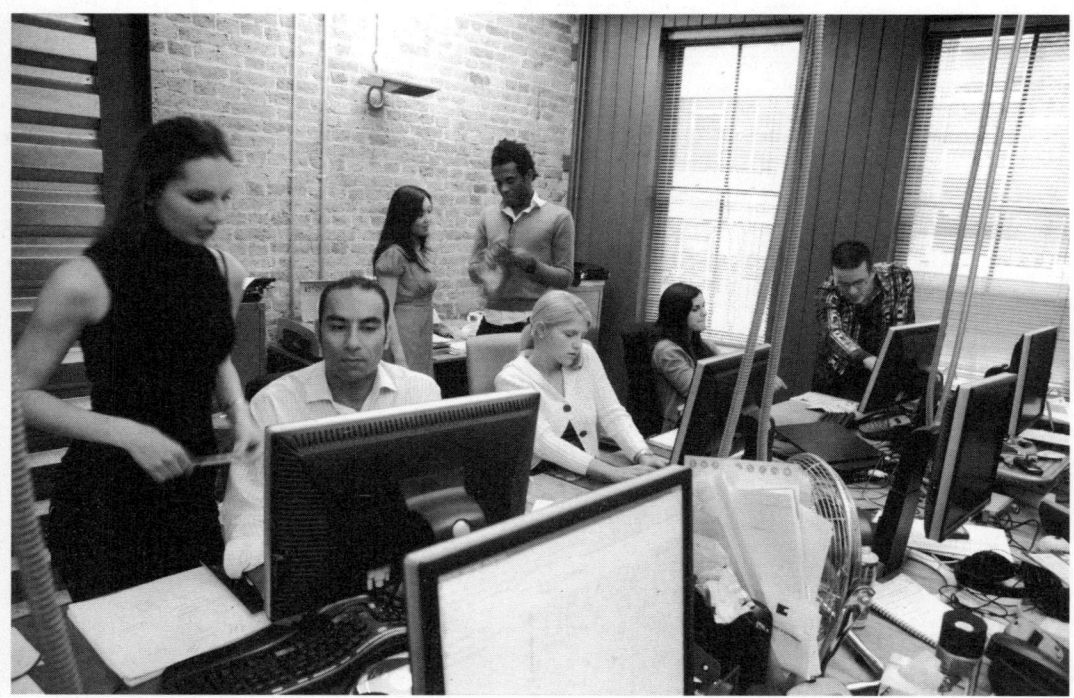

Photo 3.2 In what ways is it useful to reflect upon teams in the business world? What insights can be drawn from such attitudes to team work? Chris Schmidt/iStock.

Now that you've had a chance to consider the practice of being in a team, we turn to how team members behave when they share team values and are committed to team-working. These are key attitudes to good team-working. Remember how in chapter 1 we showed that using the model of the right attitudes to being interprofessional can lead to knowing the right thing to do and doing it right: it's the same in a team. You need those good attitudes but to know what to do and how to behave are also important.

We suggest that people in teams that work well probably do most, if not all, of the following:

- Know when to keep quiet, don't interrupt each other, speak with confidence
- Listen with care and make sure everyone can have their say
- Share their knowledge with everyone in the team
- Respect the contributions of other team members
- Actively learn and work with other team members
- Take some time to reflect on being in that team.

Relating these skills to yourself, you might like to consider these in terms of what you do and how you feel about being part of a team. In other words, try to become more self-aware about your team behaviours. For example, in a team situation have you said or done something that created an unexpected reaction in someone? When this happened were you in the best place on the model of dependency in Figure 3.1? Read Box 3.2 for some hints about self-awareness. With this in mind, we encourage you to be reflexive about how your actions impact on others – and likewise how theirs impact on you, and how these ways of behaving might affect the work that you all do together.

Box 3.2: Hints of self-awareness

According to Burnard (1997, p. 48):

... we need to know something about ourselves in order to help others. . .In a common sense sort of way. . .it would seem reasonable to assume that if we are seen as caring and sensitive in our practice, then we need to notice what it is we do.

Noticing what we do and being self-aware has two sides. It is about paying attention to what we are doing, and also reflecting on why we are doing what we do. In other words, to deliberate on what we assume, on our suppositions and our possible prejudices.

Thinking about ourselves and how we act in a team leads into the next section of this chapter, where we look at why we behave in certain ways in a team. We also look at different types of players needed to enable the whole team to be effective.

Behaviour in the team

The way we behave or act as a team member, during team meetings or in the interludes between these, clearly influences the effectiveness of the team. One clear point for interprofessional working is that each team member has the professional ability (and duty) to listen to and work with all the others in the team.

All teams are diverse: comprised of people of different ages, from different social and cultural backgrounds. Everyone has different experiences of their contact with others due to the persistence of racism, sexism, ageism and homophobia within society. It's easy for any one of us to respond in a stereotypical way about other people's social class, religion and disability. Interprofessional teams mirror this diversity and add contrasting professional perspectives acquired through different types of professional education and practice. Interprofessional working expects practitioners to be comfortable with representing their profession and their organization; and to be able to work effectively with other practitioners, often through an ability to be both leader and follower. Practitioners are expected to develop professional judgement about when to lead and when to follow; and to engage in a career-long process of scrutinizing and honing their professional judgement as they learn about, from and with others: the focus of Part II of this book.

Interprofessional team-working relies on the team members working with a range of shared principles and values: and acknowledging and accommodating some differences. This is different from allowing differences to compete in an unacknowledged way. It is different from ironing out all differences; which, even if this were feasible, is likely to diminish the creativity of the team. It is also different from subjugating all other perspectives to a dominant professional or organizational perspective.

An insight into how things can go wrong in teams with diverse members is offered by Buber (1958, p. 50). He defines two types of relationships:

> 'I–Thou': being the meeting of two people who respect each other's humanity.

And:

> 'I–It': where one person fails to recognise other people as human beings (with all that involves), but treats them as an 'object'.

This behaviour can be described as a binary: you are either one thing or the other. In practice, though, what any one person is will depend on many factors, including where they are in their career, their level of experience of working in a particular setting, who else is in the team. You can probably add more to this short list.

In the interprofessional context, we depersonalize the concepts of I–Thou and I–It, so that rather than being about individual people the concepts apply to other professions or types of work. This is a shift from being a person who would normally treat everyone else as a human being (so they are normally an I–Thou sort of person) to someone who behaves as an I–It sort of person, seeing others as from a particular profession or work setting. This results in someone from one profession (or work setting) not respecting the contribution of those from different professions (or work settings). This is, of course, why respect is considered such a key component of good team-working and essential to being interprofessional.

Developing some self-awareness about how you fit into the binary model of either I–Thou or I–It is valuable. Consider the questions in Pause Point 3.1. If you are learning in an interprofessional team, the responses of each of you to these questions would make a valuable group discussion.

Pause Point 3.1: About my prejudices

Do I have prejudices towards other professions and types of work?
What are these prejudices?
How can I overcome my prejudices?

In chapter 1 (Box 1.4), we suggested that two of the competencies needed for being interprofessional were having respect for the views of others (which may be different from your own views) and being willing to share what you know with others. We want to build on what we said about these to see how exercising these two competencies can support effective interprofessional team-working. First we discuss being respectful and then sharing knowledge.

We think that respect is one of those things that is easier to show (or not to show) to someone than it is to describe as a way of being. We had this problem with describing being interprofessional in chapter 1. Here, we want to look at what it means to be respectful with you, through the work you did in Pause Point 3.1. We have some other questions for you to think about:

- What effect do your prejudices have on others?
- How does the nature of your prejudices (what they are) influence how you interact with others?
- How has your attitude to others changed as your assumptions are set aside through knowing more about them?

Having a prejudice leads to making an assumption about someone from another profession. In turn this creates a boundary between you and them. Within their boundaries team members have assumed identities and all of this can lead to misunderstandings and ineffective team-working. Professional boundaries and identities are two things that are created by the way a profession works in its own interest. We looked at some aspects of the professions in chapter 1, so if you need to remind yourself about this go back to Box 1.3. Here our point is, as Barnett and Griffin (1997, p. 33) wrote, that professional boundaries are formed because 'Professional bodies, disciplines, departments and schools have traditionally clustered around sets of ideas and practices'.

In this way each profession is defined, bounded by its practices, its knowledge base, its philosophies and its values. The same thing happens for all types of work, whether or not any type would traditionally be called professional work. Practitioners within these boundaries assume similar identities. These are often misunderstood by those outside the boundary, hence the importance of learning about and from each other. Effective interprofessional team-working requires that these differences are recognized and worked with for an effective outcome of the team's goals and purpose. It means that sometimes our professional identity has to be put aside and we need to assume an interprofessional identity: moving from independence to interdependence and (perhaps) dependence, as in Figure 3.1.

To summarize so far . . .

We have emphasized that being interprofessional means team-working. Team-working in this way shares characteristics with working in other sorts of teams, for example, business, sports and more traditional public service delivery teams. Self-awareness and reflective practice are ways of finding out more about yourself as a team member in any of these teams.

Both identity at work and the boundaries around practice settings influence how we behave as a team member. The respect we show to others is shaped by our assumptions about identities and it influences the boundaries we put between ourselves and others. How well we share what we know with others in the team, communicating interprofessionally, is another key aspect of collaborative practice.

Interprofessional communication

Practitioners often communicate in writing by making contributions to client/patient notes, requesting assessments or tests, making referrals and so on. Spoken communication ranges from formal meetings, briefings or handovers, to informal discussions in practice settings. It may be face-to-face, by telephone or, increasingly, through a web link. Each form of communication has its own conventions, strengths and weaknesses, and practitioners must become skilled across the spectrum. This is made easier by remembering that the central purpose of communication is to progress the service user's case or management by sharing information appropriately and effectively. We look at communication again in chapters 5 and 9 to gain a deeper understanding of how practitioners share information (more or less effectively) to support their separate work and the shared interprofessional endeavour.

As the key purpose of interprofessional teams relates to decision-making (and problem-solving), the processes involved in interprofessional working comprise more than the exchange

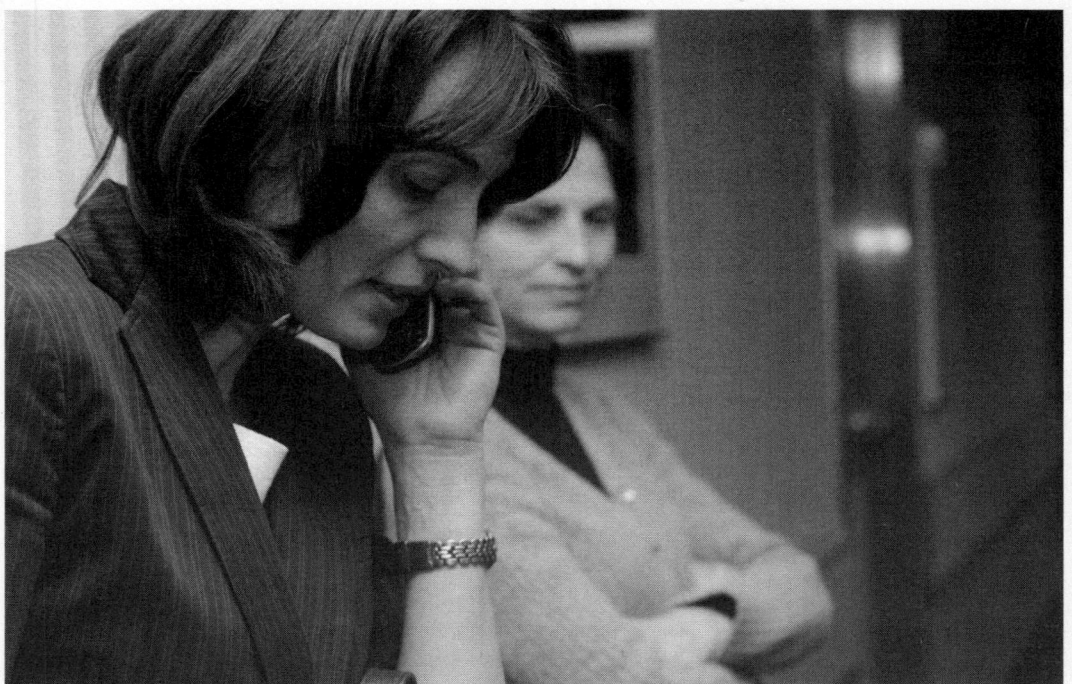

Photo 3.3 Choosing a suitable means of communication and using it effectively is a vital part of working interprofessionally; each method of communication has advantages and disadvantages – what might be the disadvantages of using a telephone in the above scene? Yarinca/ iStock.

of information between contributing practitioners. At times, possibly more often during initial team meetings, perspectives and contributions may be at odds with one another. It is important for team members to modify their inputs in light of what else is being considered. To help you manage this effectively in the team setting we suggest that you think about these transferable communication skills and how you might adapt them for yourself:

- Be an active listener; this means encouraging the other person(s) to explain fully what they mean and their needs, etc., and ensuring that the interaction is focused fully on them
- Use questions to clarify points and to make sure meanings are shared
- (Where appropriate) Be aware of body language, not only in terms of what someone is conveying to you, but also what you might be unintentionally conveying to the other person
- Become adept at giving effective and constructive feedback.

There is often a tension between what should happen and what does happen in team-working. Resolving these differences is at the heart of interprofessional team-working, with members remembering what they know about being interprofessional and being able to put this into practice. Interprofessional interactions between team members take the team's work forward and help it achieve its purpose.

If we look at the levels of interactions in an interprofessional team the explicit expression of these within a work context is often visible, for example, the application of protocols, procedures and professionally based practices. What is far less visible is how each member of the team interacts with and is affected by colleagues. When the interprofessional work is not going well, hidden agendas can be created and alternative ways are found of dealing with things. Frequently, two or three individuals informally share their thoughts and feelings. These interactions are often described pejoratively as gossip, but gossip has a purpose. It is one of the processes through which practitioners construct meanings and communicate emotion. Gossip is part of the learning process. It can be integral to how we learn our trade, and to be part of the team, as well as how we learn to be interprofessional in a team.

Gossip is also what people turn to when their team does not openly discuss important and yet contested issues. An unhappy or dysfunctional team may have members who use significant amounts of gossip as a way of expressing their views on the team and its processes. The main difficulty with gossip as a means of communication is that it is not inclusive and, consequently, it undermines full interprofessional collaboration.

Exclusive or informal conversations also take place because of the constraints of working within pre-set and different organizational structures. For example, some working patterns or timetables can result in some members of the team never being present at the same time as others. The absentees may be left out of crucial information loops, so their knowledge and skills are then missing in the service package available to the user.

Emotions within team work

Success in being a team member and taking a specific role in any team is underpinned by the need for skills, like being able to empathize with other people. You may have already met this topic in relation to how you interact with clients/patients/service users. Here we want to emphasize the importance of empathy in understanding each other in a team and to spotlight the value of emotional intelligence and emotional literacy as useful ways of thinking about our feelings. These terms are currently very popular and are used by authors such as Goleman (1997) to explore the links between the way we think and the way we feel. We would add to that the need to understand how we then act; specifically, how we behave in an interprofessional team.

We bring to our interprofessional work our knowledge, skills and attitudes, and our emotional selves. As Jaques and Salmon (2007, p. 32) write:

> Contemporary life places a premium on the ability of people to get on with each other, to be able to handle interpersonal problems rather than to avoid them, and to do so constructively and creatively.

This applies to everyone who learns and works interprofessionally. The issue is how to manage this aspect of ourselves in our interprofessional practice. Help is to hand from the notion of assessing your emotional intelligence, which Wikipedia describes as:

> **Emotional Intelligence (EI)**, often measured as an **Emotional Intelligence Quotient (EQ)**, describes an ability, capacity, or skill to perceive, assess, and manage the emotions of one's self, of others, and of groups (<http://en.wikipedia.org/wiki/Emotional_intelligence>; accessed 15 January 2008)

One model of emotional intelligence shows it having four elements: the ability to **perceive, use, understand and manage** your emotions (Mayer and Salovey 1997). Lipsett (2006) stresses the necessity for 'self awareness' and 'self-management'; i.e. managing your own emotions

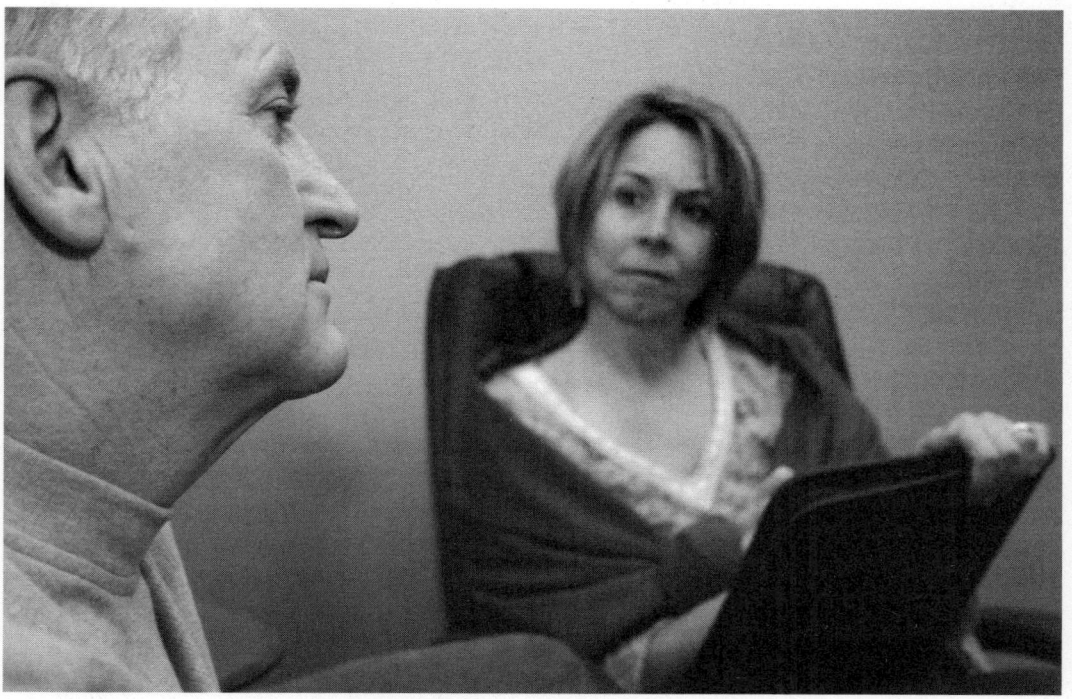

Photo 3.4 Emotional intelligence is a critical skill; it is important to be able to control one's own emotions and personal judgements so as to act in the best interest of the client or patient. Brad Killer/iStock.

so you get the best out of them. Emotional intelligence is a new and developing concept. Its appeal for people trying to identify the key elements of effective interprofessional teams lies in its link with reality. We can all remember times when our colleagues have made us feel angry, disappointed and anxious; times when our emotions have risen to the top and perhaps spilled over. Being aware of this, and learning to manage these emotions during and after team meetings, can make a positive contribution to our ability to work in an interprofessional team. Learning about this for yourself is the first step to doing the same for others. Being able to empathize or tune into the emotions of others is an important part of team-working. By understanding and/ or anticipating what colleagues need, perhaps by way of emotional support, is an asset that you can bring into your team practice.

To turn to a perspective from business, Thomson's (1998, p. 24) work on emotional capital – the feelings and beliefs that motivate people to take positive action – suggests that how we feel has as much impact on our actions as what we know. He offers what he considers to be the 'ten deadly emotions' (Box 3.3). After reading through the list of deadly emotions we suggest you do Learner Exercise 3.3.

Box 3.3: Thomson's Ten Deadly Emotions (1998)

Fear – feeling of distress, apprehension or alarm.
Anger – feeling of great annoyance or antagonism.
Apathy – lack of motivation.
Stress – mental, physical or emotional strain or tension.
Anxiety – state of uneasiness or tension.
Hostility – antagonistic or oppositional behaviour.
Envy – discontent or a begrudging feeling.
Greed – excessive desire for power or wealth.
Selfishness – lack of consideration for others.
Hatred – feeling of intense dislike.

Learner Exercise 3.3: Team work and the Ten Deadly Emotions

Look again at the notes you made for Learner Exercises 3.1 and 3.2 about teams with which you have been involved. Select one and think about one episode of team work. Make some notes that describe what the team was working on, what needed to be done, how it was approached, who was involved and what you did.

Now, using Thomson's Ten Deadly Emotions, reconsider your narrative and add, where appropriate, any emotions that also featured – your own first. You may wish to note emotions that were absent as well as those present. Were there emotions that you detected in others? Were these feelings engendered by your actions or by the action of someone else?

From the perspective of team-working, many of these emotions are often hidden – but they are there none the less. In an effective team, the members manage to resolve issues that arise from these feelings to the mutual benefit of all. One question for all those working in teams is how much effort they are willing to expend to make sure the emotional capital of the team is as effective as its professional capital. This is a demanding process and not always achieved. It adds to the complexity and challenge of being interprofessional.

The life cycle of a team

Early in this chapter we noted that many teams in community services and health care form briefly to address a particular need and then disperse to continue their separate work. However, you will also join teams which, apart from some variation in membership over time, work together over days, weeks, months and even years to provide a service or deliver a project. These teams have been observed to have a fluctuating life cycle. Tuckman's (1965, pp. 384–99) model for group development is one of the best-known descriptions of this. It has five phases – Forming, Storming, Norming, Performing and Adjourning – and teams that work together effectively go through these phases. Sometimes they enter and re-enter the phases more than once.

Forming is where the team comes together for the first time; sometimes this simply involves everyone saying who they are and where they are from and sometimes it includes deciding on tasks, etc.

Storming comes next, where the competing ideologies and/ or personalities may start to clash; this often occurs when the real work of the team starts.

The resolution of these clashes is seen as the Norming phase.

The Performing phase is when the team is working in a truly collaborative way.

Adjourning (a phase that Tuckman added later) is when the team's work is completed and they break up.

You may have worked in teams where these processes or phases happened in the sequence suggested by Tuckman. It's normal for teams to return to phases more than once. Possibly you have witnessed a team going round and round in short-circuited phases for a while and noticed that during this time very little was achieved. The interprofessional team, with its diverse dynamics, can find it challenging to achieve sufficient stability for productive work. This may be especially so with a team of practitioners who don't work together consistently, but collaborate on a case-by-case basis, or when practitioners come and go according to the needs of the service user, client or patient (as, for example, they did for Lindy in Learner Exercise 4.2 in the next chapter).

A pattern of changing team membership, varying according to the service users' needs, highlights the idea described by West (2004, p. 45) as 'team tenure'. This idea helps to remind us that a single practitioner's contribution to a patient's or client's care occurs during just part(s) of a longer journey. Colleagues from other professions and services will also join and leave the interprofessional team at points appropriate to their contributions. These transitions have an impact upon the team. After each change the team needs to re-establish shared purposes and goals alongside shared ways of knowing, discussing and deciding. The smooth, perhaps almost automatic, functioning of the team may falter for a while. It may return to one or more of the forming, storming or norming phases, described above. All members need to be actively committed to making these transitions and re-establishing effective team processes as easily and swiftly as possible. Experienced practitioners can help to smooth transitions, ensuring that the evolving team always continues to work cooperatively towards the central purpose of providing a safe, effective, efficient and compassionate service to people with evolving needs.

Short-lived *teams of the moment*, which respond to a particular problem and immediately disperse, experience highly abbreviated or missing stages of Tuckman's team processes model. For emergency response teams, the training, often aided by simulation and the accumulation of many short-lived team experiences, allows competent short-term functioning, performing without paying attention to the other phases. But this would not work if people wanted processes to evolve, perhaps in the light of new evidence or changed circumstances. Then a development process would be needed, with the team possibly going through the full range of phases described by Tuckman.

Leadership in interprofessional teams

All teams need leaders. At times this is the most senior member of staff; in other situations a leader may emerge or may be chosen by the team members based on expertise. Interprofessional teams rarely have a single leader, someone who everyone else lines up behind. This is not to say that leadership is not part of interprofessional practice, but rather to note that in settings where people work together interprofessionally leadership might well be something that changes as the service user's needs change. We pointed out in chapter 1 that health teams have traditionally been led by practitioners from high-status professions and that for twenty-first-century interprofessional working, in novel settings aimed at specific client groups, this may not be appropriate.

We now look at a more modern model of leadership called 'servant leadership' (Spears and Lawrence 2002; Neill et al. 2007). We believe this is a useful model to guide interprofessional working. It is better able to acknowledge the complexity and inherent tensions of the tasks that interprofessional teams undertake and to recognize the changing nature of the team's purpose as, for example, the needs of the service user change. The model is summarized in Box 3.4 and you will see that it puts the onus on the leading team member to understand all elements of otherness – including the 'growth of people' and 'strengthening relationships' – and of making use of this for the benefit of all.

> ## Box 3.4: A summary of servant leadership
>
> The principles of servant leadership include listening, awareness, conceptualisation, foresight, stewardship, commitment to the growth of people, and community building. Servant leaders are encouraged to build and strengthen relationships with other team members and appreciate and value the expertise and contribution of other disciplines in planning and provision of care.. . .The integration of servant leadership principles in practice has less to do with directing other people and more to do with serving their needs and in fostering the use of shared power in an effort to enhance effectiveness in the professional role. (Neill et al. 2007, pp. 426–7)

Many of the words used to describe a servant-leader link well with the key features of being interprofessional and those used to describe being a valuable member of a team. This is why being a servant-leader fits so well with being in the interprofessional team. But leaders, even leaders who take that role for a short time for a specific reason, also need leadership skills, particularly skills that:

- Encourage others to follow their lead
- Nurture team members
- Support relationships in the team
- See the work of the team generally, as a pattern or model
- Plan for the future.

Our two lists in Table 3.1 are words from the description of servant-leadership in Box 3.4. List one has those already familiar to you from reading this book; list two has words that link with the particular skills of a leader that we just discussed. By listing

Table 3.1 Servant leadership, being interprofessional and being a team member

LIST ONE	LIST TWO
listening	conceptualization
awareness	stewardship
build and strengthen relationships with other team members	foresight
	commitment to the growth of people
appreciate and value the expertise and contribution of other(s') community building	serving. . .needs
	fostering the use of shared power

these separately we are emphasizing the need for leaders of interprofessional teams to be interprofessional, to be a valuable team member as well as being a leader.

Team members as team types

Returning to our earlier theme that the quality of team work depends upon the quality of contributions from team members, we now want to look at how an effective team needs its members to function in complementary ways. The following section aims to start you thinking about what type of team member you are. What knowledge and skills do you bring to the team in addition to those related to your practice? What aspects of your personality are relevant to your work as a team member? Learner Exercise 3.4 uses the Belbin Team Role Types Model as a way to explore, and possibly experiment with, your team member activities.

First, a word of explanation about this sort of exercise, which is often linked to personality profiling devices. There are many profiling devices, all of which have different purposes and most can only be administered by trained practitioners, usually psychologists. This is not the place for a rigorous investigation into your personality type. What we offer is a simple and well-used exercise that can offer ways

---

Learner Exercise 3.4: Finding out about team types

1. Think back to a specific team activity that you have been involved in. Write a summary of your activities in the team: think about what you did, what sort of role you had in completing the work of the team, how you behaved towards the tasks of the team. You can do this by describing positive and negative behaviours.
2. Look at the Belbin Team Role Types in Table 3.2 and try to match yourself to them, using the way you were involved in the activity you described. One way of doing this is to award yourself stars where there is a match (either for your contributions or for allowable weaknesses). The more you think there is a match, the greater the number of stars. You might find that more than one section describes your *type* or that large elements do not chime with your views of yourself – this is OK. The purpose of the exercise is for you to try to look at your behaviours from an outside perspective.
3. Now discuss what other members of the team found and see from your comparisons how the team was constructed. Was there a balance of team types, were too many of you trying to coordinate, was anybody a completer-finisher, how many were specialists – those sort of questions will help you to assess why the team is successful or maybe why it is not, so far, working as well as it could be.
4. Reflect on what you found out about yourself during this task. What does the exercise tell you about putting together a team?

of thinking about your own behaviour and team personality, and those of others, in relation to a standardized format.

The people who originally designed the Belbin Team Role Type tool are happy for it to be reproduced and used by other people, and it can be fun! It offers some insights into the varieties of personalities that occur in teams (identified by a particular group of psychologists). It's not intended to be an exhaustive list and give you definitive answers. It is an aide-memoir to support your reflections about team types. Learner Exercise 3.4 sets out what to do to find your team type and Table 3.1 helps you to compare what you found with a set of standard types. Like other learner exercises in this book, you can do this by yourself or, preferably, do it with others from an interprofessional team.

In Table 3.2 the descriptions of some of the team types hint that people of this type have some of the skills necessary to be a leader in the team. For example, the coordinator type is said to make a good chairperson, the shaper has drive and the team-worker averts friction.

Table 3.2 Belbin's team-type roles from <http://www.belbin.com/belbin-team-roles.htm> (accessed 26 June 2007). Reproduced with kind permission from Belbin Associates

Team-Role Type	Contributions	Allowable Weaknesses
PLANT	Creative, imaginative, unorthodox. Solves difficult problems.	Ignores incidentals. Too pre-occupied to communicate effectively.
COORDINATOR	Mature, confident, a good chairperson. Clarifies goals, promotes decision-making, delegates well.	Can often be seen as manipulative. Offloads personal work.
MONITOR EVALUATOR	Sober, strategic and discerning. Sees all options. Judges accurately.	Lacks drive and ability to inspire others.
IMPLEMENTER	Disciplined, reliable, conservative and efficient. Turns ideas into practical actions.	Somewhat inflexible. Slow to respond to new possibilities.
COMPLETER FINISHER	Painstaking, conscientious, anxious. Searches out errors and omissions. Delivers on time.	Inclined to worry unduly. Reluctant to delegate.
RESOURCE INVESTIGATOR	Extrovert, enthusiastic, communicative. Explores opportunities. Develops contacts.	Over-optimistic. Loses interest once initial enthusiasm has passed.
SHAPER	Challenging, dynamic, thrives on pressure. The drive and courage to overcome obstacles.	Prone to provocation. Offends people's feelings.
TEAMWORKER	Co-operative, mild, perceptive and diplomatic. Listens, builds, averts friction.	Indecisive in crunch situations.
SPECIALIST	Single-minded, self-starting, dedicated. Provides knowledge and skills in rare supply.	Prone to provocation. Offends people's feelings.

Most people can act in more than one team-type role. It is important to remember that a balanced team is one in which people between them cover all roles, and in this way it is more likely to function well. If your team appears to lack, for example, an implementer; consider whether this is a role you could fulfil. If not, who could you identify to fill this gap?

Types and purposes of teams

Moving on from the types of personalities that meld their efforts to produce effective team work, we look next at the different types and purposes of teams. All teams, including interprofessional teams, have a different purpose and their working processes will differ according to this purpose. For example, working with one or two colleagues from other work settings for a specific client can lead to participating in an interprofessional case conference. From this you may be asked to join an interprofessional working group to look at more general issues related to similar clients in the future. There is more on this is chapter 5. Here we want to draw your attention to ways in which some of the purposes and characteristics of different teams have been described by people who study teams (Boxes 3.5 and 3.6). Their work relates mainly to the business sector, but we believe it aids understanding of teams within community and health services too. The types and characteristics we have included in the boxes below are those which appear most relevant to the sector we are writing about. You can read more about other types of, and purposes of, teams in the references we have given.

Box 3.5: Different types of teams according to purpose

Advice and involvement teams, e.g., management decision-making committees, quality control groups, staff involvement groups.

Production and service teams, e.g., assembly teams, maintenance, record-keeping and evaluation, imaging departments and laboratories processing diagnostic tests.

Project development teams, e.g., research teams and service development teams.

Action and negotiation teams, e.g., surgical teams, rapid response units and trade union negotiating teams.

(adapted from West 2004, pp. 18–19)

Cross-functional teams – these are teams with staff from the same hierarchical level, but different functional areas within an organization or even between organizations.

Quality Circles – these teams are concerned with improving quality and effectiveness, stressing participative objective-setting.

(Adapted from McKenna 2000, p. 330)

Box 3.6: Characteristics of teams which influence teamwork

Degree of permanence – a stroke rehabilitation team may work together for years, sharing the progress of many patients, but a resuscitation team may only be together for the minutes that elapse while they care for one patient.

Emphasis on skills/competence development – breast cancer care teams must continually develop their skills in response to new evidence, new drugs and technologies, changing attitudes towards palliative care, quality of life decisions, patient and family involvement; whereas decision-making committees usually have little emphasis on their skill development and more on knowledge management.

Genuine autonomy and influence – many service delivery teams have relatively little autonomy and influence whereas top management teams are powerful.

Level of task from routine through to strategic – many activities within screening services are fairly routine, well-defined and often somewhat automated; investment in new or upgraded screening services demands strategic planning and negotiation with multiple stakeholders.

(Adapted from West 2004, pp. 18–19)

Pause Point 3.2: Reflection on the teams I belong to

Think about the workplace teams you know.

How many of the team types in Box 3.5 are represented?
Now focus on a specific interprofessional team that you have been part of.
Which of the characteristics in Box 3.6 apply to this team?

Pause Point 3.2 is designed for you to reflect on how some of the interprofessional and other teams you are familiar with relate to the team purposes and characteristics outlined in Boxes 3.5 and 3.6. Box 3.7 has suggestions for further reading about how teams work.

Box 3.7: Further reading about how teams work

Katzenbach, J. R. and Smith, D. K. (1993) *The Wisdom of Teams: Creating the High-performance Organisation*. Boston: Harvard Business School.
This book offers insights into the key question about teams and includes explorations into when and why team-working might be appropriate.

West, M. (2004) *Effective Teamwork: Practical Lessons from Organisational Research*. Oxford: Blackwell.
This book gives a comprehensive account of teams and team-working – from the perspectives of both theory and practice – and also offers a wide variety of useful educational tasks to help develop understandings.

To conclude

Practitioners have always had to interact with others in the course of their work. However, the consciousness and accountability for professional action in collaborative working is now in much sharper focus. This has led to the need to increase our understanding of our interprofessional actions and duties and our ability to carry them out.

We believe that being interprofessional and working collaboratively needs something extra adding to the usual attributes ascribed to (other) teams. One of these is the need for a different approach to leadership. The shift from the tradition of defined roles and leaders to the modern context, where the service delivery is more complex and many service users have multiple needs, has changed initial and continuing education programmes. Understanding how teams function, knowing about your role in the team, what team types you are, and what skills are valuable, is necessary if you are going to be part of an effective team.

We wrote in the opening chapters of the book about the knowledge, skills and attitudes you need to be interprofessional. We hope that you now feel more able to work interprofessionally. But it is foolish to think that the work and effectiveness of an interprofessional team is solely influenced by the capability of each member to be interprofessional. Collaborative work is also shaped by its purpose and context – agencies and organizations that provide public services, their policies and procedures, and the wider political and social arena. All these influence collaborative working.

The way the modern UK public sector is organized means it is impossible to always meet user needs from the services and resources offered by just one agency; and we feel the same is true in most other countries. Many of the people who use health and social care services have complex needs. You will read in chapter 8 how some service users are best served by collaborative working across the statutory, community, private and voluntary sectors. The reality of practising interprofessionally means collaborating with colleagues, with the service user, and with carers across multiple and diverse agencies. This is complex and happens in different ways depending upon the needs of service users and the range of services available. In the next chapter we will look at some extended examples that illustrate this complexity in different areas of practice.

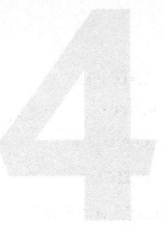

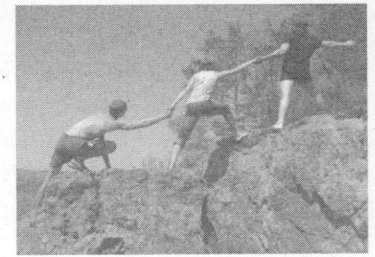

Being Interprofessional
in Complex Situations

Whatever you do will be insignificant, but it is very important that you do it.

Mahatma Gandhi

What you will read in this chapter

This chapter extends what we said in chapter 3 about teams, team-working and team membership by discussing being interprofessional and collaborating with others in complex situations. We explored teams in some depth because team-working of various types is the means by which *being interprofessional* is achieved. Being an effective team member and understanding how teams work are not ends in themselves. Rather, they are the means towards executing your professional role well within a complex service delivery organization. Increasingly, this is also often about collaborating with colleagues from other service delivery organizations from the statutory, community, voluntary and private sector providers (about which we say more in chapter 8).

We now want to look at interprofessional working from three perspectives which we believe underpin efforts to deliver good services through collaboration with others:

- Responding to service users in complex situations
- Responding to past failures or guarding against perceived risks
- Collaborative practice and professionalism.

We examine these perspectives largely through case-based material. The cases are all grounded in the experiences of real people and are complex enough to have features from each of the categories listed above. We have chosen not to simplify them to the point where each only addresses the particular heading under which it is placed. This means you can move backwards and forwards through the chapter, drawing ideas from each real-life example for each section of discussion and each learner exercise.

Responding to service users in complex situations

We could have written a whole book about this! Instead we use three multifaceted examples to draw out the main points about collaborative working – as the necessary response to complexity and challenge. First, we look at an example of long-term work with sexually exploited young people. These people can be hard to help and robust multi-agency work is needed (see the quote from Harper and Scott, below). Staff in schools, youth offending teams, the police and health care are those most likely to have initial contact with young people at risk because early indictors include children going missing from school, home or care, or the diagnosis of a sexually transmitted disease (Harper and Scott 2005). But practitioners are often reluctant to identify the risk, or have not received adequate training to do this.

> The key message is to be proactive: sexual exploitation will remain hidden if services simply wait for it to reveal itself as a problem locally. All agencies working with young people – including schools, health services, the police and social services – need to be aware of the indicators of risk and be prepared to act. (Harper and Scott 2005, p. 2)

Inter-agency protocols that ensure a collaborative response are helpful, but even then the work can be difficult and needs to be long term. Out of forty-five local agencies interviewed in one study of three south London boroughs, forty-one agencies believed they had knowledge of children and young people known or suspected to be sexually exploited (Liabo et al. 2000). In the quote below, someone from a Social Services Department describes how one pimp, who had groomed numerous girls (some as young as twelve or thirteen) was first identified.

> It was first picked up by one of the child-care coordinators. There were three young people. . .all in children's homes at the time. The social worker spent a great deal of time talking to one of the young people. . .and a year later, she was willing to tell us much more. . .By then we were aware that there were about 14–15 youngsters. . .(Liabo et al. 2000, p.3)

There has been confusion in the past about whether the young people involved are victims or offenders – police guidance now states that they should be seen as young people in need. However, at first sight, some of the young people seem to have entered sexual exploitation voluntarily, and they can be wary of practitioners. It takes time to develop trust.

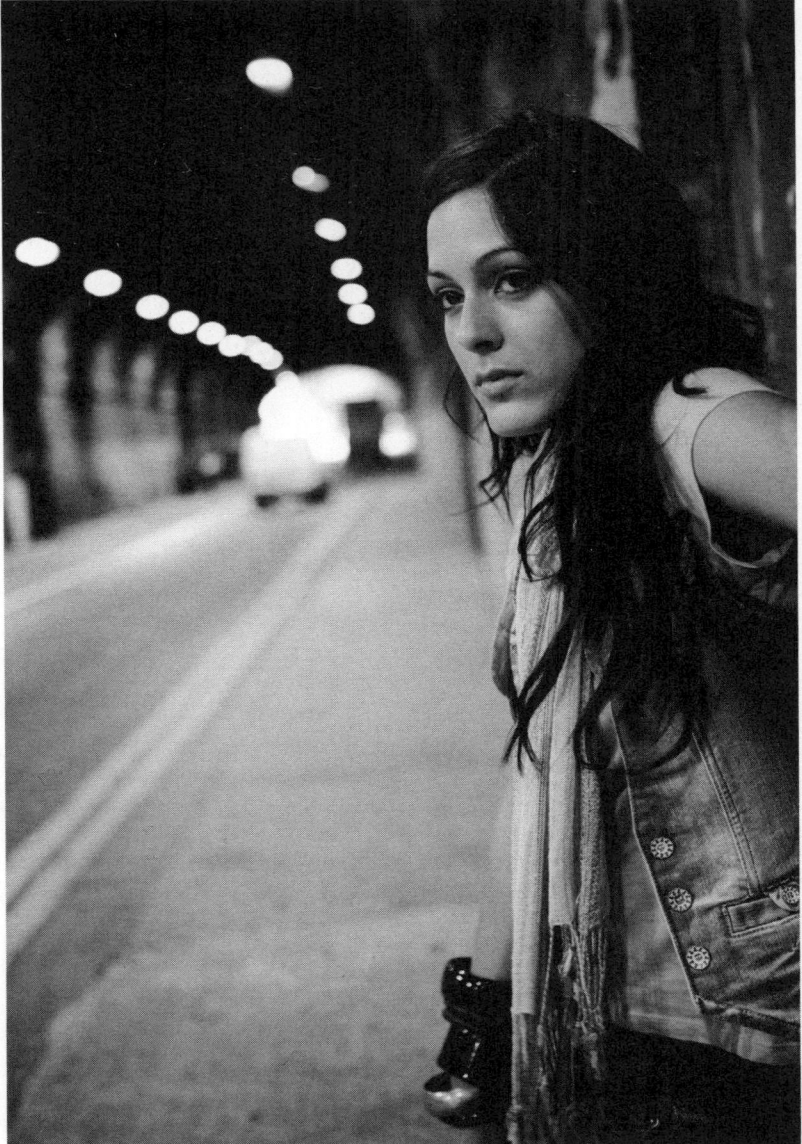

Photo 4.1 Who might be involved in keeping young vulnerable people away from prostitution? What different approaches and attitudes might each professional have? Chris Schmidt/iStock.

Liabo et al. (2000) identified some of the needs of young people involved in sexual exploitation as:

- Accommodation, financial support and safety
- Substance misuse services
- Education
- Sexual health and sex education
- Emotional support.

As the list above shows, a number of service providers are involved in preventing sexual exploitation, protecting sexually exploited young people and prosecuting those who perpetrate this abuse (Harper and Scott 2005). However, priorities and time scales differ between agencies. The police must look to prosecuting offenders as the main means of protecting vulnerable people. Social services, schools and other education providers, mental health services, substance misuse services and voluntary networks, to name but a few, need to engage in long-term work with both victims and offenders, focusing on prevention and support.

Young people who have grown up in the care system are one of the groups of young people particularly at risk (see the quotes below, from Liabo et al., and Harper and Scott). Peer pressure, material rewards, drug use, fear of coercers, lack of self-esteem, denial of their situation and lack of good alternatives can make it difficult for young people to want to move away from their involvement in prostitution. Intensive practical, emotional and therapeutic support can be crucial in breaking ties.

> A lot of the time kids aren't able to say 'I'm worth more than that.' They just aren't able to (as a result of) some of the stuff that happens at home or wherever. (Liabo et al 2000, p. 36)

> Many of the young people who became at risk of sexual exploitation in adolescence had been failed earlier in their lives so improving the quality of services, particularly social services is another aspect of prevention. (Harper and Scott 2005, p. 6)

The extract in Learner Exercise 4.1 is adapted from a case study in a national report by Barnado's – *Whose Daughter Next?* (1998, p. 25) – which outlined legislative and practice challenges to dealing with sexual exploitation in the UK. This exercise is designed to help you think through some issues related to meeting the needs of vulnerable young people in relation to the many agencies that may need to be involved in their care. As well as reflecting on your own position in relation to D's situation (next page), try to discuss this or other similarly complex situations in a small interprofessional group.

Other groups of service users with complex needs can be equally hard to reach and help. They include people with substance misuse problems, people who are homeless or who move very frequently, victims of domestic violence and other groups at high risk of social exclusion, such as asylum seekers and refugees. Another group are people of all ages whose desire or need for services conflicts with the wishes of their families; they include:

- People with physical or mental impairments and whose desire for independence is in conflict with the wishes of their families
- People who live very cloistered lives within families or small communities and lack the language skills or daily freedom required to access services independently

- Children whose parents or guardians do not agree with the assessments and recommendations of practitioners and service agencies.

Learner Exercise 4.1: Inter-agency and interprofessional responses in complex situations

D is a fifteen-year-old girl who had been in regular contact with the project for two months. She began to have only intermittent contact (i.e., once a week), which gave staff cause for concern. The next occasion D used the project she had a counselling session about her safety. It emerged that she was being locked in a room by her *boyfriend* for security. She said, "He's changed. I remember going for a walk in the park and we drew a love heart on the wall and put our names on it – it's still there now. . .." After a thorough discussion of her safety, D admitted her life was/may be in danger . . .

Here are some questions to help you with your reflections on the issues raised:

Which agencies and what types of practitioner might now be able to help D?
How can they best coordinate their complementary contributions?
Who should lead this response?
Do you think any of the participating agencies will have conflicting priorities that may hamper smooth inter-agency collaboration?
What do you think might happen in terms of tensions, working at cross-purposes and emergent gaps?
What should happen if D is too frightened to seek help at this point and asks the counsellor to forget all about what she has just said?

Pause Point 4.1: Working with people with complex needs

In which aspects of your practice are you likely to be aware of potential service users with complex needs who, due to their circumstances or the nature of their needs, are difficult to help?

- Who would it be helpful to collaborate with in these circumstances?
- Do you have the skills that you need?
- With whom might you work to strengthen your skills and how will you arrange this?

Focusing on journeys through services

Learning and working with patients/clients/service users and user-focused services are the main subjects of chapter 6. Here, using the idea that the service user takes a journey as s/he uses services, we want to show:

(a) the interprofessional team in the context of complex (and that often means inter-agency) team-working; and

(b) team changes in response to the changing needs of the service user.

The concept that someone using public services is on a journey is most often used in health care. Mapping this journey serves different purposes. It can be a way of:

- Seeing how the care needs of a person vary with time and to solve problems by being able to picture what is happening along a timeline (Lavender and Walker 2003)
- Gaining a better understanding of the patient's experience and of promoting their voice about their experiences, especially people with chronic diseases (British Medical Journal 2004 and Langgartner et al. 2005).

In Case Study 4.1 we describe the journey through care for Lindy, a person whose care needs have changed over time. Learner Exercise 4.2 asks you to look at her journey and think about how her care has been delivered. As for similar exercises earlier in this book, we suggest that you first do this exercise by yourself and then with other students in the interprofessional team.

Case Study 4.1

19 July 2007

Yesterday Lindy was watching the Ladies' Bowls Team; they lost but it was good fun and she enjoyed playing the piano for the evening's singing in the clubhouse after the match. She forgot that she had an appointment with the chiropodist. Today she is having lunch out with her family to celebrate her eighty-second birthday. She tells them that the food is almost as good as the meals on wheels she has every day.

Tomorrow is the day her home help comes so she will have company for a while. Lindy misses her small dog but knows how impractical it is for her to have a pet now. In the afternoon she will have her monthly blood pressure check with the practice nurse and see her doctor about her memory problems.

20 July 2007

Lindy is on a stretcher in the corridor of her local district hospital, waiting for an X-Ray to confirm that she has broken her leg. Her daughter tells the radiographer that although her mum's name is Rosalind she is always called Lindy and she is rather deaf. Later that night, during surgery to pin the fracture, Lindy has a stroke. After two months in the stroke rehabilitation unit she is able to speak again, although she muddles up pronouns. Even after doing exercises the speech and language therapist taught her, Lindy struggles to eat solid food. She no longer likes the taste of tea or coffee. Despite a lot of physiotherapy she can't walk at all. She never regains use of her left hand and spends hours learning to write with her right hand. Her hearing aid has been lost and no one seems to realize that a new one would make a difference to her collaboration with the staff. Lindy is eventually transferred to a nursing home run by a private company; her notes stay in the hospital. Her house is sold and her family fit a few special pieces of furniture into her new tiny room. They learn about fees for nursing home care from the home's social services liaison worker.

July 2008

Lindy still asks when she is going home. She has a new hearing aid but the battery always needs changing and no one seems to think it's their job to do that sort of task. Her son has asked the volunteer who brings his dog in for Lindy and the other residents to stroke if he would change the battery, but it's not his job either. Lindy has lost a lot of weight and needs to be hoisted every time she is moved. This is painful for her and sometimes she shouts at the health-care assistants. Every day at 10 a.m. and 3 p.m. she is asked if she would like a cup of tea. She doesn't answer the question any more.

The staff can't cope with Lindy's behaviour so she is referred to the community geriatric psychiatrist. After the psychiatrist's visit no one is sure what to do. The note in the day book about a prescription for anti-depressants refers to someone called Rosalind. There is no one in the home with that name.

Learner Exercise 4.2: Care services during a patient's journey

Lindy's increasing dependence on care means that she has been looked after by a number of practitioners from different agencies. Her family have been involved and visit her when they can and local friends see her regularly.

First, make a list of the services and practitioners involved in caring for Lindy in 2007–8. Make some notes about how this changed during the year. Have all her needs been responded to?

Second, can you identify any gaps in the service she is receiving in 2008? Could Lindy's care be improved by staff working collaboratively? Is there anyone who is not being included in the team caring for Lindy? Would including them help Lindy?

Finally, think into the future for Lindy. What other sorts of care services might she and her family need? Who else might be involved?

Anyone using social care and health services will meet new practitioners as the route of their journey changes. Different types of practitioners may come into the team, while some members of the team may leave. That new member may be you. You may find yourself working interprofessionally with new team members who you need to learn about, from, and then with, so that services are effective. You may also find yourself working in more than one interprofessional team and in teams that span different organizations. You may be based in one organization and expected to provide services or advice in another. For example, suppose your social work practice is in local authority children's services and you are consulted about a child presently in hospital care. This means you will join a team of other practitioners primarily based in health care, such as children's nurses, paediatricians, play specialists, teachers managing the interface between hospital education and normal school, and so on. Like you, other practitioners in the team, for example, a clinical psychologist, may have a different work base. To contribute most effectively to this team during your period of membership (team tenure – look back to chapter 3), you will need to be aware of the work of teams who have contributed prior to your involvement and mindful of the teams likely to take over in the future. In this way we can shape our practice more to the user's experiences.

Pause Point 4.2: Relating team work in theory to practice

Look back to chapter 3, particularly the sections on:

- Effective team-working
- The life cycle of a team
- Leadership in interprofessional teams.

Think about the general principles outlined in these sections and how they relate to the specific case studies in this chapter.

Another practice area where care is provided by a wide range of practitioners is palliative (also called end-of-life) care. Here is another example of where providing effective services is complex and can be challenging. The World Health Organisation (WHO) definition of palliative care is shown in Box 4.1 and WHO offers additional points that relate specifically to children (see <http://www.who.int/en>).

Palliative care is probably more likely to be seen as a care approach for people like Sally who have cancer (Case Study 4.2). But it is also suitable for people with any disease or condition that cannot be cured, particularly when they have distressing symptoms that need to be alleviated. The statutory, voluntary and private sectors are all important providers of palliative care, often in hospices and by specialist palliative care teams. For Sally, hospice care was also available at home, but that can vary depending on where you live.

Palliative care teams consist of practitioners from a wide range of backgrounds to meet a person's physical, psychological and social needs at the end of his or her life. Take a look at all the different practitioners involved in Sally and her family's care in Case Study 4.2. In palliative care, practitioners with different professional and

Box 4.1: Definition of palliative care (WHO 2008)

Palliative care:

Provides relief from pain and other distressing symptoms.

Affirms life and regards dying as a normal process.

Intends neither to hasten nor postpone death.

Integrates the psychological and spiritual aspects of patient care.

Offers a support system to help patients live as actively as possible until death.

Offers a support system to help the family cope during the patient's illness and at the time of their own bereavement.

Uses a team approach to address the needs of patients and their families, including bereavement counselling, if indicated.

Will enhance quality of life, and may also positively influence the course of illness.

Is applicable early in the course of illness, in conjunction with other therapies that are intended to prolong life, such as chemotherapy or radiation therapy, and includes those investigations needed to better understand and manage distressing clinical complications.

Case Study 4.2

Sally has just spent another two weeks in her local hospice. The medical and nursing staff have managed to get her pain under control. She and her partner feel confident about her medication regime and know that her family doctor, the district nurses and the local pharmacist are on hand to give advice if necessary. A specialist nurse has been helping to care for her wounds and Sally is confident that these won't seep or smell with the new dressings. Her family and friends have promised to help out with meals and shopping, and her children came to the meeting at the hospice about her discharge. They want Mum at home. It's important for her and the children to have as much time as possible together. The teachers at their schools know that Mum is coming home and that they might miss some lessons.

This time in the hospice Sally talked to the chaplain about how she always planned to die at home. A major bleed from her wound and severe pain had been so frightening. She was afraid her family wouldn't cope and didn't want to be a burden. Talking it through helped her realize that they are a strong family with a strong network of friends. She hadn't realized that a chaplain would just listen; she was so relieved that there was no pressure to say a prayer! Just before she left, Sally and her partner spoke to the social worker about applying for a government allowance. They are now much less worried about their financial situation.

Sally is now at home. The hospice-in-the-community team are looking after her. She feels included in all the normal comings and goings of family life and content that she is where she always wanted to be at the end of her life.

ethical frameworks work collaboratively. Seeking consensus from many points of view in difficult situations can be challenging. The patient and their family and friends are important members of the team. Team decisions in these situations are often complex, and successful team-working needs practitioners who can work well interprofessionally.

We discuss learning and working with service users in detail in chapter 6. Here, we want to recognize that the wishes and experiences of people using services (in this case palliative care services) are a central concern of professional and interprofessional practice (see the quote from the National Institute for Health and Clinical Excellence (NICE), below). Sally was helped to spend the end of her life at home by different practitioners working together to help her achieve her wish.

> Studies have consistently shown that, in addition to receiving best treatments, patients want to be treated as individuals, with dignity and respect, and to have their voices heard in decisions about treatment and care. (National Institute for Health and Clinical Excellence (NICE) 2004, p. 3)

Box 4.2 sets out some features that patient/client-focused services need to be mindful of, adapted from work done for people with cancer (NICE 2004, p. 5). We have adapted them to cover situations where interprofessional collaborative working is important. Our point is that working in the ways indicated in Box 4.2 is not straightforward; it is, however, necessary and practitioners are expected to have the skills to work in these types of teams.

In complex and difficult team situations, using effective communication skills and showing respect for all others are ways to maintain team coherence and keep the focus on the common

---

Box 4.2: Features of patient/client-focused services

Services need to recognize that:

Individual patients/clients have different needs at different phases of their illness and life, and services should be responsive to their needs.

Families and carers need support during the patient/client's life and in bereavement.

Families and other carers have a central role in providing support to patients.

Some patients/clients need a range of specialist services.

It is important to forge partnerships between patients/clients and carers and health and social care practitioners to achieve best outcomes.

Effective multi-agency and interprofessional team-working depends on interprofessional partnerships.

Services need to be ethically and culturally sensitive.

purpose of the team (return to chapter 1 if you need to review these aspects of being interprofessional). Where there is tension between the needs and wishes of people in receipt of palliative care and the needs and wishes of their families, end-of-life care needs a breadth of knowledge, flexibly applied, with the ability to move beyond stereotypes. Emotional intelligence (see chapter 3) is important here too.

For those in need of palliative care, the decision about which people are in the team will depend on the patient's needs at a particular time. For people who have cancer there is often a Macmillan nurse (and you may want to visit their website to find out more: <www.macmillan.org.uk/Get_Support/About_Macmillan_Nurses/>). As patients/clients journey through palliative care, practitioners will join or leave their care team. As we discussed in chapter 3, in these circumstances leadership of the team may be different for different phases of work. This means the most appropriate practitioner or service leads and coordinates others – traditional hierarchies should be irrelevant. If leadership and coordination (not necessarily a single role) are to pass from person to person or agency to agency, then 'handing over the baton', to use a metaphor from athletics, needs to be explicit so that everyone notices this has occurred. There is no place for batons to be dropped and not picked up.

Pause Point 4.3: Your role in palliative care

Think about your own area of professional practice in relation to the definition of palliative care in Box 4.1.

Which facets of that definition are you most likely to encounter in your routine work?
What sort of contribution are you likely to be able to make?
What knowledge, skills and attitudes will be required to do this well?
Are you well prepared? Or do you need to learn, practise and observe more?

You might also like to take time to consider, from the work you have been involved with, if your client/patient recognizes who is/are the leader(s) for their care – and do the rest of those involved concur?

Responding to past failures and currently perceived risks

The second perspective on interprofessional collaboration we wish to discuss is the way in which professionals and agencies respond to past failures or currently perceived risks. As for the section above, we could have written a whole book on responses to past failures.

But instead we take a shorter route through some key principles, drawing mainly from an extended example in the field of improving child protection. Other areas where high-profile incidents have prompted responses that, among other measures, stress the need for effective interprofessional and inter-agency communication and collaboration include mental health and children's surgery. See, for example, Blom-Cooper (1995), Parker and McCulloch (1999), and Kennedy et al. (2001) on the issues raised at Bristol Royal Infirmary (the Bristol Royal Infirmary Inquiry <www.bristol-inquiry.org.uk>). In focusing on one case (Box 4.3), we are able to trace some new ways of working, from their origins in failings identified during a public inquiry, to calls for policy and practice changes that are now enshrined in UK law.

Box 4.3: Improving services for children in need: lessons from the inquiry into the death of Victoria Climbié

Victoria Climbié died, aged eight, after months of cruelty from her aunt and the aunt's partner, who were subsequently convicted of her murder. Victoria had been seen by a large number of practitioners and agencies (see Box 9.5 later in this book) but all had failed to rescue her. A public enquiry, led by Lord Laming, explored what happened during the months leading up to her death (Laming 2003). Amongst other things, the enquiry revealed a lack of collaboration by police, health care and social services staff responsible for assessing Victoria's well-being, as well as poor inter-agency working arrangements.

Box 4.4: Two recommendations from Laming (2003)

1 . . . establish a 'common language' for use across all agencies to help those agencies to identify who they are concerned about, why they are concerned, who is best placed to respond to those concerns, and what outcome is being sought from any planned response.
2 Newly created local Management Boards for Services to Children and Families should be required to ensure training on an inter-agency basis is provided. The effectiveness of this should be evaluated by the government inspectorates. Staff working in the relevant agencies should be required to demonstrate that their practice with respect to inter-agency working is up to date by successfully completing appropriate training courses.

The inquiry report (Box 4.4) emphasized a need for practitioners to communicate differently and more effectively; to receive and apply appropriate training; and for effective oversight of services provided. Take a moment to read Pause Point 4.4 and think about these issues in relation to your own practice.

Pause Point 4.4: Focus on your area of practice

Are there any concerns about the potential for differences in the use of language and communication procedures between practitioners from different specialities and agencies to create misunderstanding or gaps in the service provided?
Do practitioners have appropriate training for inter-agency working?
Who has oversight in order to identify and remedy any shortcomings?

Victoria Climbié's death was neither the first nor the last potentially preventable death to be investigated; but its severity meant that it prompted policy-makers and practitioners into action. Reorganization of children's services followed Lord Laming's report and drew on a number of the report's other recommendations. We return to this when we write about information sharing in chapter 9. Here, we look at some government responses to Laming (2003) and (in the following section) how three professional bodies collaboratively contributed to new ways of working in children's services.

The UK government's response to the Laming Report

The UK government's response to Lord Laming's Report is known as the Every Child Matters agenda. This is enacted in UK law through the Children Act (2004). There is a lot of information about this on the Every Child Matters website: <http://www.everychildmatters.gov. uk>. Initially, the government presented a Green Paper, *Every Child Matters – Early Intervention and Effective Protection* (DfES 2003). As the quote below shows, this recognized the difficulties experienced by the multiple agencies responsible for providing children with effective support and care.

> Children's needs are complex and rarely fit neatly with one set of organisational boundaries. For instance, a child with behavioural problems due to parental neglect may be considered a child with special educational needs by the Local Education Authority, a 'child in need' by the social services, or having a conduct disorder by a child and adolescent mental health team. . .The categories around which services are organised are overlapping, fluid and, in some cases, blurred. (Department for Education & Skills 2003, p. 68)

All papers related to the Every Child Matters agenda highlight the need to improve collaboration and information sharing between agencies as central to improving practice. There is also the requirement for practitioners to integrate better, especially in work to identify at-risk children. Better integration only happens when members of staff are capable of being interprofessional and have leadership and followership skills. In this way, the lead professional

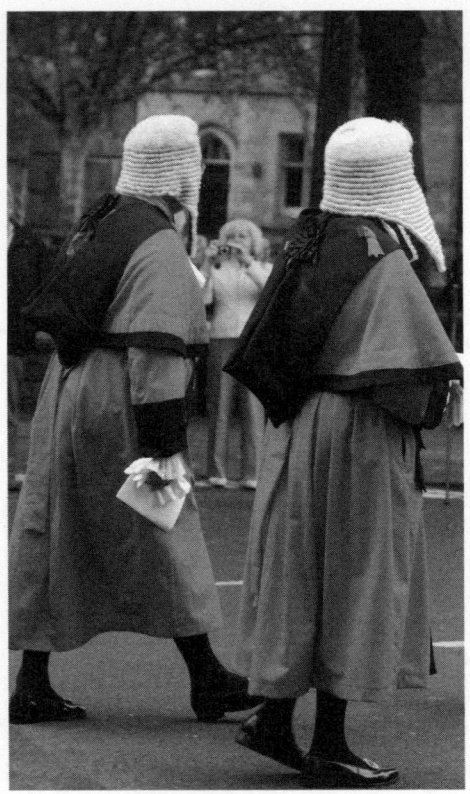

Photo 4.2 Practice in all areas is ultimately driven by law; effective communication between practitioners and lawmakers is extremely important and probably one of the most difficult forms of interprofessional communication. William Murphy/iStock.

(and others) in children's services can positively influence the services provided by reducing overlap and inconsistency (DfES 2004, pp. 2–4).

These policy-led solutions alone do not guarantee effective services. The attitudes of practitioners to new ways of working in children's services, which included seeking more permeable boundaries between agencies, are of considerable influence. Perhaps now is a good time to remind yourself about the attitudes we set out for being interprofessional in chapter 1. As you study towards entering the working world, take a moment to reflect on how your practice fits into this more flexible and responsive agenda that is ultimately driven by UK law.

There are many different agencies charged with delivering education, care and support for children. Box 4.5 shows services or individuals that a child might be in contact with through his/her journey from infancy to adulthood. The potential number of organizations and agencies, both statutory and informal, for any given child is large. Their scope is wide-ranging. This is not to suggest that all these groups are in direct contact with each other, but to alert you to the scale of potential interprofessional interactions a single child could activate. It's not difficult to see why effective interprofessional practice across agencies that collaborate with each other determines the provision of the optimal children's services.

Government policies say 'that developing networks across universal and specialist professions can strengthen interprofessional relationships and trust' (DfES 2003, p. 63). We suggest that an important part of professional practice involves each practitioner taking individual responsibility for looking at how to develop and maintain interprofessional networks to support service users' best interests. Take a moment to read Pause Point 4.5 for some insight

Box 4.5: Agencies and practitioners involved in children's services

Local Education Authorities: schools, educational welfare, youth services, special educational needs, educational psychology, child care, early years education.

Social Services: assessment services for children in need – such as family support, foster care, residential care, adoption services, child care, advocacy services, child protection and services for care leavers, social workers.

Community and Acute Health Services: general practitioners, health visitors, community paediatric services, drug action teams, teenage pregnancy coordinators, child and adolescent mental health services, speech and language therapy.

Children and young people may also engage with youth and community workers, school nurses, home visitors, volunteers and mentors, housing officers, the police, voluntary sector staff.

They may also come into contact with religious organizations, sports and sport associations, youth groups and organizations that support specific recreational and social activities.

Pause Point 4.5: Developing professional networks for working with children and young people

Think of a child or young person that you have worked with. List how many of the groups and practitioners in Box 4.5 they will have come into contact with.

Sort these according to the four main professional groupings overseeing the provision of support and care for children:

Social services
Health services
Education
Police and criminal justice services.

Now consider which agency and what colleagues on your list you need to learn more about, who you can learn from, and how best you can learn with colleagues to ensure the service you provide is as good as you would like it to be.

into developing interprofessional networks around your practice with a child or young person. We now turn to how the collaborative practice we discussed above is integral to your practice and professional practice generally.

Collaborative practice and professionalism

We wrote in the opening chapters of the book about the knowledge, skills and attitudes you need to be interprofessional. We hope that you now feel more able to work interprofessionally. But it is foolish to think that the work and effectiveness of an interprofessional team is solely influenced by the capability of each member to be interprofessional. Already in this chapter it has become clear that collaborative work is also shaped by its purpose and context. Collaborative working is influenced by agencies and organizations that provide public services, alongside their policies and procedures, and the wider political and social arena.

The way the modern UK public sector is organized means it is impossible to always meet user needs from the services and resources offered by just one agency (we feel the same is probably true in most other countries). Many of the people who use health and social care services have complex needs. The reality of practising interprofessionally means collaborating with colleagues, with the service user, and with carers across multiple and diverse agencies. This happens in all areas of practice, but in different ways depending upon the needs of service users and the range of services available. This means it is inevitable that some of your work as a professional practitioner will involve being interprofessional. It involves working collaboratively in different ways.

Professional bodies also have a role in creating interprofessional practitioners. These organizations primarily exist for practitioners of a particular profession; they work on behalf of their members. Sometimes called the 'professional project', this can lead to an inward focus on its practitioners by the professional body, rather than focusing on the user of the professional services that their members offer. Of course, at times, it is necessary and right for professional bodies to prioritize their members. But doing this exclusively is counter to the modern climate of involving the customer, with marketization, that we wrote about in chapter 2. As we discussed, in the twenty-first century, professional bodies need to be interprofessional: learning and working about, from and with each other.

Some professional bodies have played a part in helping their members with their interprofessional working. To illustrate this, we stay with services for children to show how three of them worked together to enhance services. The General Social Care Council, the General Teaching Council for England, and the Nursing and

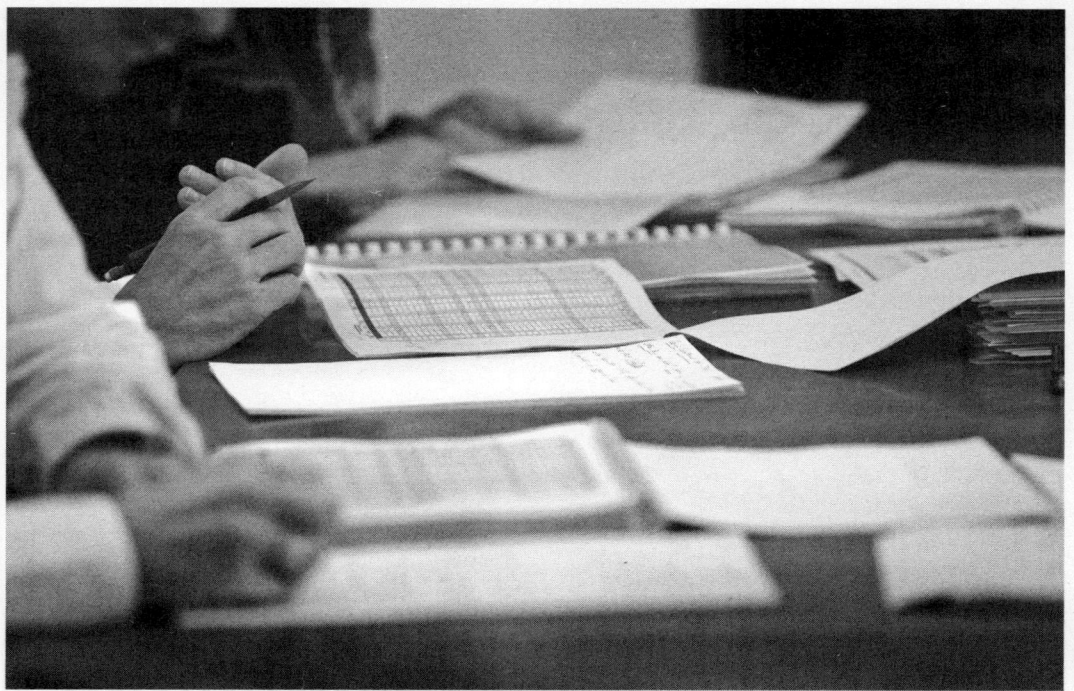

Photo 4.3 When drafting codes of practice, professional bodies need to strike a balance between protecting the interests of their own members and working interprofessionally for the good of service users. Nikada/iStock.

Midwifery Council, agreed a statement of values to underpin their working. (Box 4.5 is an excerpt relating to interprofessional work with colleagues.) Their statement was also developed in consultation with service users (children and families) and many other organizations. We feel the final statement would be applicable to all children's practitioners – see our list of these in Box 4.6.

As Box 4.7 shows, as part of the Every Child Matters agenda, the term 'children's practitioner' has been created and is applied to everyone who works with children. This means that all practitioners working with children and young people are identified as being children's practitioners at the same time as being a particular type of practitioner (e.g., a social worker, teacher or nurse) and, of course, being interprofessional team members. In Learner Exercise 4.3 we encourage you to think through the implications of this new term.

Another aspect relating to the professional development of collaborative practice is interprofessional development and training. This is an area of work usually undertaken by education providers and staff familiar with current practice and policy. This probably includes the interprofessional programmes you participate in as pre-registration or undergraduate students or in your continued professional development.

Box 4.6: Interprofessional work by three professional bodies

The statement below of interprofessional values underpinning work with children and young people by the General Social Care Council, the General Teaching Council for England, and the Nursing and Midwifery Council: Interprofessional work with colleagues is available from <http://www.nmc-uk.org.uk/aArticle.aspx?ArticleID=2326> (accessed 9 September 2008).

Children's practitioners value the contribution that a range of colleagues make to children's lives, and form effective relationships across the children's workforce. Their inter-professional practice is based on a willingness to bring their own expertise to bear on the pursuit of shared goals for children, and a respect for the expertise of others.

Practitioners recognise that children and families, and colleagues, value transparency and reliability, and strive to make sure that processes, roles, goals and resources are clear.

Practitioners involved in inter-professional work recognise the need to be clear about lines of communication, management and accountability as these may be more complex than in their specialist setting.

They uphold the standards and values of their own professions in their inter-professional work. They understand that sharing responsibility for children's outcomes does not mean acting beyond their competence or responsibilities.

They are committed to taking action if safety or standards are compromised, whether that means alerting their own manager/employer or another appropriate authority.

Children's practitioners understand that the knowledge, understanding and skills for inter-professional work may differ from those in their own specialism and they are committed to professional learning in this area as well as in their own field, through training and engagement with research and other evidence.

They are committed to reflecting on and improving their inter-professional practice, and to applying their inter-professional learning to their specialist work with children.

Work with children can be emotionally demanding, and children's practitioners are sensitive to and supportive of each others' well-being.

In the planning and implementation of initial and continuing interprofessional programmes we require education and service institutions to work together, to jointly fund initiatives and to bring their staff together to facilitate and support students' learning. Needless to say, this is logistically difficult, and often involves working across multiple sites, merging diverse timetables of classroom and service learning for cohorts of students. Indeed, the issues of working collaboratively within the professional workplace are mirrored exactly in the education provider sector, often requiring precisely the same principles and skills to overcome the challenges, shared goals, effective communication, flexibility and mutual respect.

Box 4.7: The range of practitioners who have new multi-agency roles in children's services

Children's centre coordinator
Clinical psychologist
Educational psychologist
Education welfare officer
Family support worker
Headteacher and all staff, primary school
Headteacher and all staff, secondary school
Health visitor
Learning mentor
Personal adviser
Play worker
Police officer
Probation officer, youth offending team
Social worker
Substance misuse service manager
Young offender institution case worker
Youth offending team member (drugs and alcohol)

Learner Exercise 4.3: Names and roles for working with children

What might be the impact on a practitioner of having different identities?
    What are the advantages and disadvantages of using one name for a person who works with children for:

(a) children and their families
(b) staff
(c) organizations?

Finally, in this chapter we want to mention interprofessional working where much of the formality we outlined in chapter 3 is missing. Mostly, members of an interprofessional team would say that there is a team and their work is collaborative. But this is not always the case. Sometimes staff work collaboratively without formally thinking of themselves as a team, and they can appear and function in an almost ad hoc way. This is not ideal as it may make it much more difficult for the team to recognize the way it works, and especially to relate to what are known as team development processes.

    What is the problem with people not recognizing themselves as part of a team? When we look in practice at any type of collaborative working, we can see there is often a tension between what should happen and what does happen. From the perspective of being interprofessional, resolving these differences is at the heart of team-working – with members understanding they are part of a team, remembering what they know about being interprofessional and being able to put this into practice. It is the interprofessional interactions between team members that takes the work of the team forward and helps it achieve its purpose. So, not to see yourself as part of the team may also mean that you don't feel problem resolution is part of your work either.

The types of interactions in the interprofessional team fall into two essential categories – the formal and the informal. The formal is demonstrated through the application of protocols, procedures and professionally based practices. But, as we mentioned in chapter 3, what is far less visible is the informal, that is, the processes through which each member of the team interacts with and is affected by colleagues. When interprofessional work is not going well, hidden agendas can be created and alternative (separate) ways are found for dealing with things, which do not necessarily include all members of the team. Such communication, because it was not inclusive, can consequently undermine full interprofessional collaboration. In these situations it is important to understand that our duty of care also includes each team member and ensuring that each member feels included in the team.

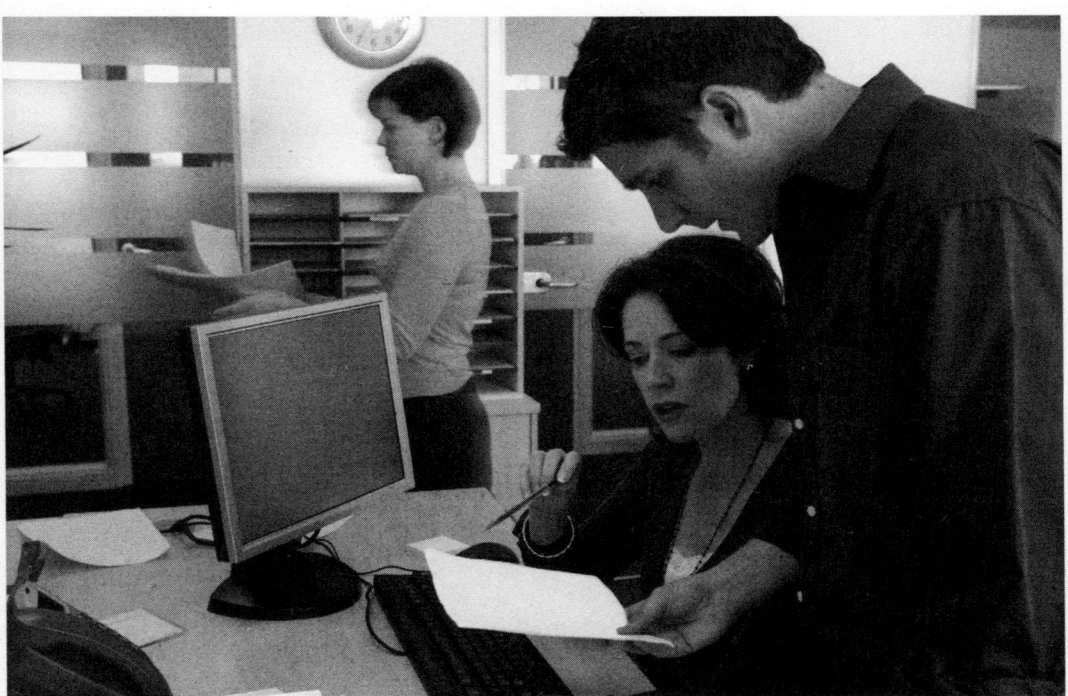

Photo 4.4 It is important that teams are inclusive; while passing on information on an ad hoc basis is sometimes necessary, make sure information is shared appropriately with all members of the team to avoid potential problems. Marcus Clackson/iStock.

To conclude

This final chapter of Part I, on the nature of being interprofessional and working collaboratively in a team, has been looking at the real, complex and challenging world of service delivery. Surrounding individual practitioners with their interprofessional competency are layers of interpersonal, team and agency processes to be dealt with. There is potential for things to go wrong. We believe that being interprofessional is important in all circumstances, in all work and in all agencies, if errors are to be kept as low as is humanly possible and service outcomes are to be maximized for all users.

Part II

About, From and With ...

In Part I we looked at the nature of being interprofessional and working as part of a team in the context of collaborative organizations. For most practitioners a commitment to work collaboratively with service users, carers and colleagues, within and beyond their immediate team, arises from internally held values and attitudes: that is, from each person's unique perspective on what it means to be a professional, how to act interprofessionally and how to provide good care or good services through collaborative working. Evidence indicates that this leads to improvement in care and services for service users (see, for example, Simmonds et al. 2001; Holland et al. 2005; Malone et al. 2007).

In Part II we examine more closely the multifaceted nature of collaboration and highlight some of the consequences of sub-optimal collaboration. The interprofessional practice of individuals sits within multiple, overlapping frameworks that are sometimes in tension. We believe that learning about these tensions and where they arise from is a vital part of the process of learning to work with others to moderate them.

In the following four chapters we examine interprofessional collaboration with colleagues, service users and carers, and look at collaboration across the statutory, community and voluntary and private sectors. All four chapters have in common the premise that learning about, from and with others is a means towards improving user and provider satisfaction with publicly funded services.

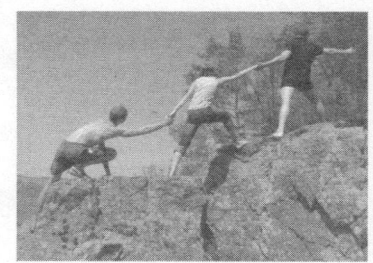

5

Learning About, From and With Other Practitioners

The only true wisdom is in knowing you know nothing.

Socrates

What you will read in this chapter

This book is about *being interprofessional* because we believe that interprofessional collaboration is the only viable way to deliver adequate services, let alone the high-quality services to which practitioners and service users aspire. The case studies throughout the book, particularly the ones about Timothy and Casey, illustrate the need for a commitment to interprofessional collaboration. *Being interprofessional* is a way of thinking and a way of working that practitioners *learn* and *refine* over time. In this chapter we focus on this continuing learning process and, specifically, on the ways we all learn about, from and with each other. We explore reflection as a learning tool and referral as a key aspect of working with colleagues.

Career-long learning and professional development, including interprofessional learning, begins during initial professional qualification. It accelerates throughout the time you spend as a newly qualified practitioner. It continues as a personal quest for improvement that is rooted in practitioners' professionalism and desire to do the best they can for service users. Learning to be interprofessional requires us to appraise our current expertise and current context. Acting professionally means doing this with honesty and a mindset that celebrates what is good. It asks that we identify specific areas for improvement and take manageably small steps towards improvement. The examples in this chapter illustrate this process.

It is worth noting that, while we are focusing here on learning about *being interprofessional*, the process illustrated is the same for learning many other things that contribute to being a competent practitioner, valued by others and, within yourself, appropriately proud of your expertise and contributions to care. It applies to learning within your own profession, discipline or services just as much as it applies to learning about, from and with practitioners from other disciplines and other service agencies.

Active learning

Learning is an active process: it happens when we *engage* with problems, challenges, new ideas or unfamiliar practices and through this engagement learn new things. Reading, listening, thinking and writing are the bedrock of much of our learning, as a look at the different ways learning has been defined (Box 5.1) shows.

It is the thinking and writing (which forces thinking) that really matter because they are the *active* parts which lead to learning. We can all read and listen passively without learning or absorbing anything, but that is not a particularly good use of time; neither does it lead to the sort of leaning that stays deeply within us. Learner Exercise 5.1 is designed to help you understand more about how the active–passive model applies to your practice of reading.

Learning by doing things and working out how to improve what we do is really important. This is why initial professional education includes so many practical activities, either real or as some form of simulation of reality. Once you are qualified, doing things within your practitioner role becomes the main focus of your professional life. But it's not just about *doing*: it's much more about the way things are done. Doing things thoughtfully ensures that learning can continue throughout your career. The examples presented shortly illustrate how an inexperienced practitioner begins to work more thoughtfully, learning from experience and from working with others. Participation in daily work, accompanied by increasingly rigorous thinking to guide subsequent participation, is the foundation of the active learning in these examples.

Box 5.1: Definitions of learning

- A change of behaviour as result of experience or practice
- Acquisition of knowledge
- Knowledge gained through study
- To gain knowledge of, or skill in, something through study, teaching, instruction or experience
- The process of gaining knowledge
- A process, by which behaviour is changed, shaped or controlled
- The individual process of constructing understanding based on experience from a wide range of sources.

(Adapted from Pritchard 2005)

Learner Exercise 5.1: Active learning and its application

1 Stop and think about how you are using this book. Is it passive or active?
2 Have you actively chosen which parts to read and which parts to skip over? Were your choices good ones?
3 Have you thought about how to apply the things you are reading about? For example:

- Making small changes to your *behaviour* in particular contexts in the near future
- Incorporating what you have read and thought about into a written piece of work.

This could be an essay, a personal development plan entry, a professional portfolio entry, an application for funding or other resources, a paper for managers or colleagues addressing proposed service or process improvements, or an educational resource to help others.

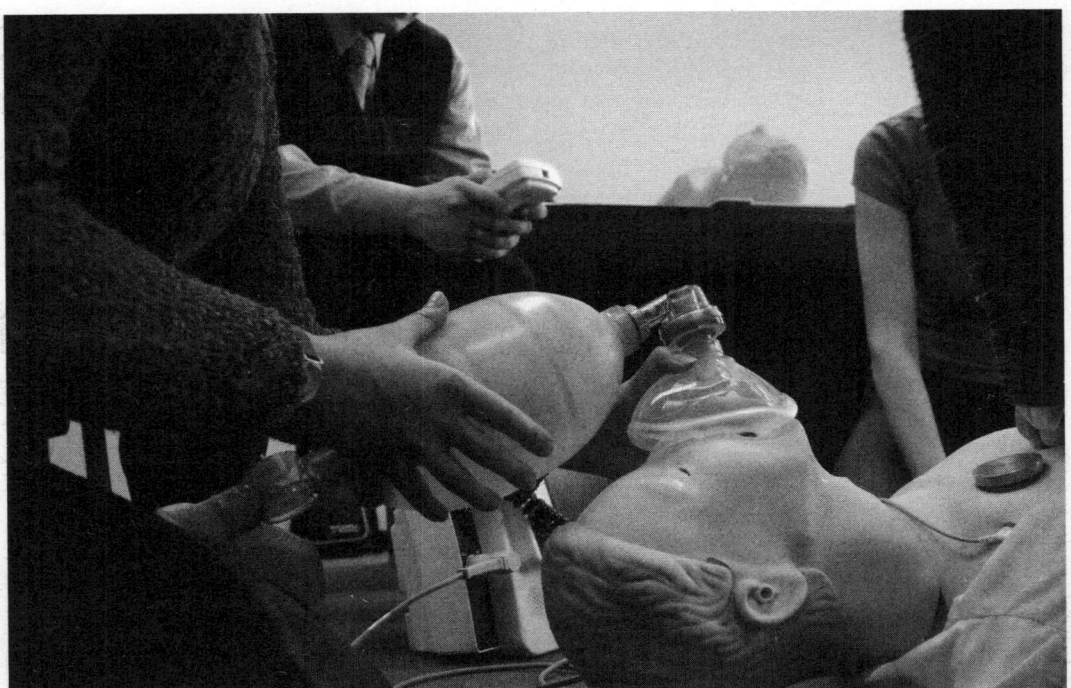

Photo 5.1 Learning by *doing* is a crucial aspect of learning, such as simulations and hands-on practice in CPR training. art-4-art/ iStock.

What we learn enables us to help service users more effectively and allows us to be useful members of interprofessional teams. In chapter 1 we wrote how being interprofessional means knowing what to do, having the skills to do it and doing it with the right attitudes.

We feel this is worthy of a reminder here as we focus on the learning process, a reminder that what we learn as we go about our daily work should include:

- Knowledge – *what* is known, including sufficient knowledge about the basis and limits of professional practice for your own profession or work setting and for those professions with whose practitioners you would expect to interact; and organizational procedures and protocols
- Skills – *how to* do things, including technical profession-specific skills, organizing yourself and others, communicating effectively, sharing (collaborating), anticipating and reviewing
- Attitudes – *having a particular frame of mind*, including patient/ client-centredness, valuing collaboration and so on.

If you remain alert to the possibility of learning you will find that almost every week you will hear, read or see something that makes you think or question, provides a new insight or shows you what you need to learn next. We suggest at this point you do Learner Exercise 5.2, which has some questions to help you consider the ways you identify and use opportunities for learning. You can do the exercise alone but also try it in a small interprofessional group. Take time to think about the differences that came out of doing the exercise with an interprofessional team.

It is the process of continually learning, developing and refining your practice that makes professional life satisfying. Sometimes the prevailing context or climate, for example, national and local priorities, the environment you work in, resource constraints and pressures, plus your own reactions (in the form of attitudes and behaviour) combine to produce a phase of activity that neglects learning. You get into a routine of doing the same thing over and

---

Learner Exercise 5.2: Identifying and using learning opportunities

Think back over the last week or so and remember something you have learnt. This might be from the news, a documentary, the Internet, a conversation, a presentation, private reading, undertaking a task set by others, your daily work or social life.

Why do you remember this particular thing?

What did you (or someone else) do that changed passive seeing or hearing into active learning?

What does this tell you about other opportunities for learning or engaging with challenges?

Do you find yourself calling to mind moments when opportunities for active learning were missed?

Can you think of ways to reduce the number of missed moments in the future?

over, and this leaves you feeling less and less satisfied or motivated. This type of stagnation is very bad for your professional and personal well-being. You can't always change your context, at least not in the short term. You have a great deal of control about the attitude you adopt and often more control than you think about ways of behaving in any context. So aim to be active: try always to keep learning and developing. The satisfaction and career rewards this brings will be good for you; and your well-being will radiate out and improve the quality of life for others.

It is easy to think that active learning needs to be something big and impressive or conducted in a special place. It doesn't. Individuals and teams learn all the time because they identify *problems* they want to solve. Here, *problem* denotes a gap between what you know now and what you think you need to know; or any gap between what is happening now and what you think should be happening. The gaps you identify are not necessarily large and the problems are not necessarily intractable. They are just challenges with which we engage and through this engagement learn new things.

Learning about, from and with others

Most of the time we don't learn in isolation but through some form of social interaction. For this reason our focus now is on learning about, from and with practitioners. This fits well with our overarching theme of *being interprofessional*, but it is wider than this. It is important not to overlook the importance of learning with, from and about service users, *expert patients*, carers, voluntary workers, advocates and activists. All these people are stakeholders in the services we provide, but they don't sit comfortably under the term 'practitioners'. These groups receive some attention within the examples in this chapter but are considered in greater depth elsewhere; particularly chapters 6, 7 and 8. Neither do we wish to downplay the importance of learning in other ways besides our interactions with others – for example, from good-quality books, research reports and summaries, journalism, appropriate Internet resources, local audit results and so on. These sources extend and complement what we learn from interactions with people.

Throughout your working life you will learn from people around you and draw that learning into your own professional practice. This is more noticeable when you are a student, newly qualified, or in a new job or role. Everyone recognizes you as a learner. You are acutely aware of how little you know in comparison with more experienced colleagues and service users. The vividness of this process fades with time but we should remain alert and ensure its continuation. Another change of role or environment temporarily puts us back to the status of newcomer. For a while we (again) become more aware of learning about, from and with others. This is one of the reasons why changing roles or environment is both challenging and invigorating.

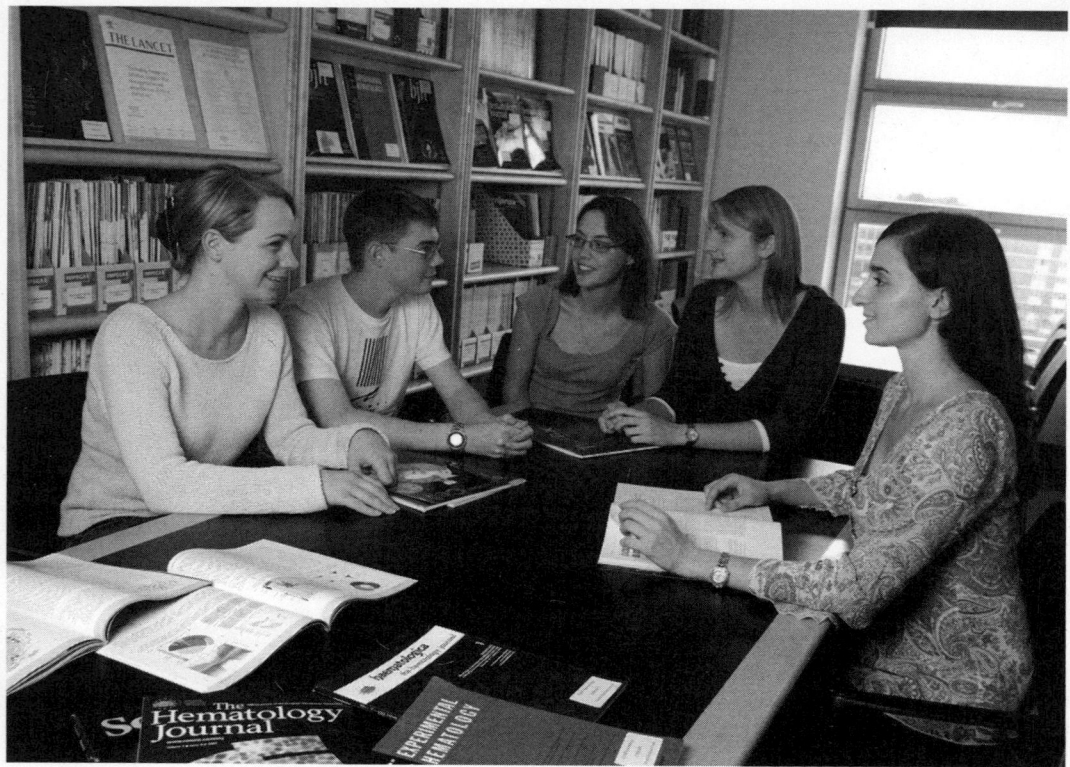

Photo 5.2 A journal club; journals and research reports are also very important learning tools. © Stephen Bond.

Learning *from* others includes observing, listening and questioning to find out how they do certain things and deciding what you should emulate or adapt in your own practice. You will adopt a critical stance. This means sifting what you see and hear, not necessarily taking things at face value and checking for applicability in your own practice. Of course, adopting a critical stance is not the same thing as criticizing others: what they do makes sense to them even if you disagree and want to try to change their mind or behaviour.

Learning from others also includes learning *about* what they do, why they do these things and why they do them in specific ways. You learn how their ways of thinking about the world underpin their daily actions and decisions. Put another way, it's learning by you about the models and theories they use and the values they adopt as they put these into practice. This learning will be all the better if it is not just one-way (from and about others) but shared. This means adopting a collaborative state of mind and collaborative actions that help all participants to develop their thinking, deepen their understanding and refine ways of doing things – learning *with* others.

In the following sections we demonstrate the reality of learning about, from and with others with a scenario constructed from many years' experience of helping novice professionals. The case study is presented as a series of scenes that you can perhaps imagine as short film clips. The I speaking to us is a character formed of an amalgam of several people's real experiences. Between each scene there is a reflection on learning built around a key issue, and some responses, to help you think about this issue for the practitioner. The scenario illustrates rapid active leaning in response to experiences at work. Due to the central character's lack of experience, much of the learning is reactive; in other words, it happens in order to 'fix' something or to solve a pressing problem. The opposite is planned or proactive learning, when you anticipate what you need to know before taking action. One of our aims here is that you will have a better understanding of the challenges of reactive learning and the benefits of proactive learning.

Case Study 5.1: (Re)active learning from and about others (and self)

Scene 1

I am newly qualified and in my first job. Reviewing my caseload, I think that a particular client is likely to benefit considerably from seeing a physiotherapist. Indeed, I hope that if the physiotherapist can improve this client's mobility some of the problems that I am currently trying to address may recede, perhaps even disappear, so I will have less work to do. Prior learning from university, pre-qualification work experience and everyday life mean that I feel reasonably confident about what physiotherapists do and that a physiotherapist could help a client such as mine. I'll broach it with the client when we meet later today.

At this point, try to anticipate what problem-solving (learning) will happen for this practitioner through this referral. Of course, this will depend upon the working context and factors such as what has been learnt so far about this client's condition, circumstances and priorities, as well as the local provision of physiotherapy services, referral practices and so on. If this scenario is outside your own experience then take this as an opportunity to fill some of the gaps in what you know, from others in the interprofessional team.

Case Study 5.1 continued

Scene 2

My client and her carer are quite enthusiastic about the possible improvements I describe. They ask about the length of the waiting list, where the appointments will be and whether there will be any help with transport. I feel foolish. I admit I don't know any of these things but undertake to find out.

Already the inexperienced practitioner has learnt that an apparently simple intervention, in this case suggesting referral to another practitioner, needs far better preparation – at least until s/he has sufficient work experience to have acquired a secure grasp of the relevant knowledge and skills. The unanticipated need for more thorough preparation has created additional work in needing to relay answers to the client and the embarrassing experience has slightly undermined her/his professional confidence. This is unfortunate when the starting premise was that this intervention may be a way to simultaneously provide good care and reduce the current workload.

Case Study 5.1 continued

Scene 3

After seeing another two clients I settle down with my follow-up 'to do' list. As well as finding out the answers to a number of questions, I have to progress this physiotherapy referral. I don't know which form to use. A passing colleague shows me where to find the form, wisely adding that I should not try to do the referral alone if this is the first one I've done. I need help from my supervisor or mentor.

My mentor is not impressed. Lines of accountability, the care plans of other members of the multidisciplinary team, budget issues and professional etiquette all mean that I should have checked things with others *before* broaching the physiotherapy referral with this client. My mentor also points out that I have paid very little attention to finding out what is important to this client and carer, or to soliciting the views of colleagues. Without sufficient knowledge about the priorities of others I won't know how reasonable my chosen priority is.

Scene 3 shows that it was sensible (and, it would appear, surprisingly easy) to seek ad hoc help from a passing colleague, rather than struggle on and probably layer new errors on top of those already committed through lack of preparation. The response redirected the inexperienced practitioner to a mentor with a formal role in helping newcomers to function safely and effectively in their new work environment by providing advice and guidance, answering questions and pointing out relevant resources – including other people who can help. Mentors are important in supporting the learning of anyone undertaking a new role or entering a new environment, not just for newly qualified practitioners. Experienced practitioners often learn to seek informal mentorship from their colleagues when they take on new tasks and roles, or move to a new environment. The allocation of a formal mentor is more important for trainees, newly qualified staff and anyone making a big transition in their work.

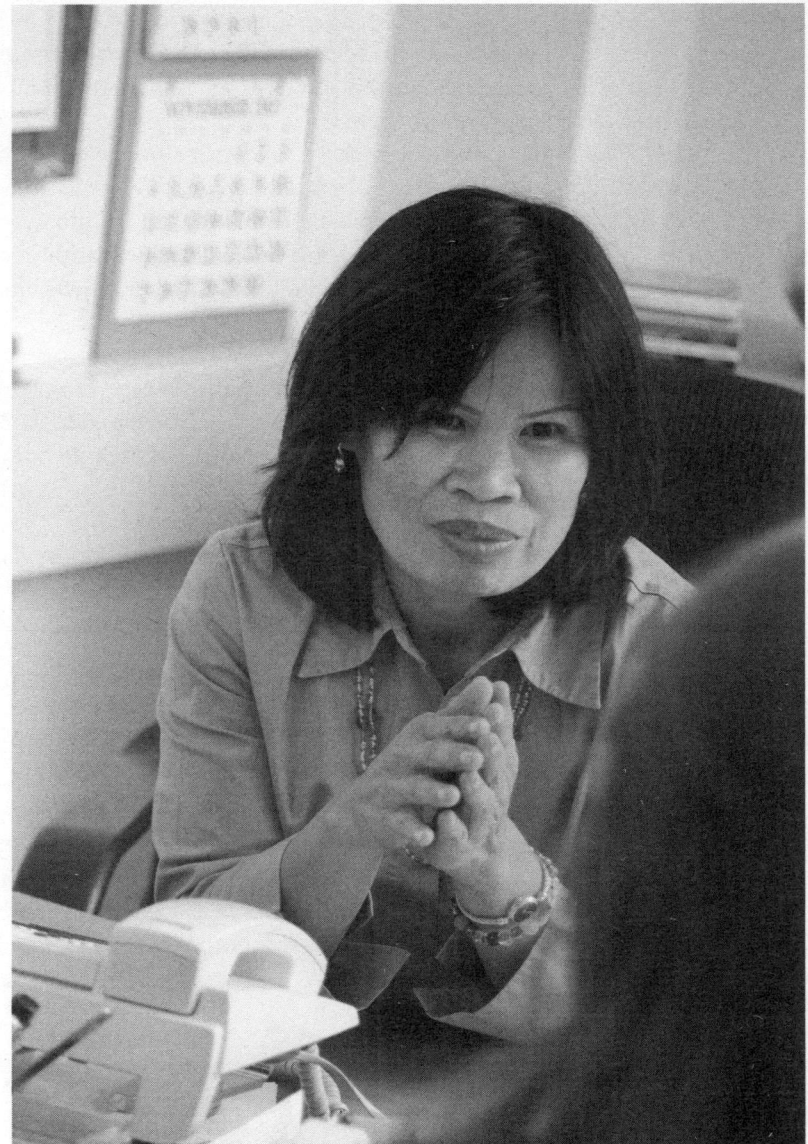

Photo 5.3 Mentors are important in supporting the learning of anyone undertaking a new role or entering a new environment. Willie B. Thomas/iStock.

Case Study 5.1 continued

Scene 4

Once dismay and anger subsided, my mentor helped me to retrieve the situation. She told me some of the things I was trying to find out. She showed me the team's shared directory of forms and procedures, and printed out the flow-chart about making referrals. We rehearsed how I was going to apologize to the colleague who should have been involved at an earlier stage and ask him if we could now discuss this client's needs.

Later that afternoon she helped me to identify more clearly what I know well enough to undertake without support and what I still need help with. Most importantly, she gently showed me a few things that I didn't even realize I didn't know. We also discussed reactive and proactive learning: something to be thinking about as my caseload increases and I take responsibility for clients with different needs.

I had known from the beginning that this was her role. I sensed that it was a role she enjoyed. But I had been in too much of a rush to make a noticeable difference to this client's management and had neglected to work through the possibilities and pitfalls. The result was certainly noticeable but not for the right reasons!

My mentor does not have time to discuss every new thing that I do. I now know that I need to think harder about which things might be more complicated than they appear at first sight and prioritize seeking support with these.

Here we can see a skilful and enthusiastic mentor at work. Immediate learning needs are met and longer-term ones are highlighted. The inexperienced practitioner has been supported and has learnt a considerable amount. This includes some new practice-related knowledge and awareness that people in this work environment will generally respond positively when asked for help. In addition, there was rehearsal of the tricky communication ahead. We can also see the inexperienced practitioner becoming more able to evaluate his or her own knowledge, skills and behaviour, as well as developing a more appropriate attitude towards seeking help and team-working.

Case Study 5.1 continued

Scene 5

I was dreading initiating a conversation with the colleague I should have involved earlier, but it went quite well really. Apparently I need to accept that while physiotherapy is likely to improve mobility for this particular client, making a worthwhile improvement to their quality of life, other issues mean that there may be more pressing priorities. It's anticipated that there will be ongoing needs in the areas I am already addressing.

Learning from this early work experience was certainly active. Now I realize that, unfortunately, most was reactive rather than proactive. I was reacting to a chain of events that I had unwittingly triggered. Happily, none were dangerous but some were certainly embarrassing. I really regret that I may have raised false hopes for this client and carer. I was genuinely trying to provide good care but I did not know enough at that time.

Proactive learning to enable good care would have involved thinking through the whole episode in advance and gathering relevant information and advice before intervening. I can see the importance of making better use of the mentor role that has been provided to support me. I also learnt from the generally nurturing and helpful responses when I asked various members of the team for help.

I am trying to store memories of how I felt when I realized I was getting out of my depth and how the various responses helped me to move out of this worrying position. I hope to be able to recall these memories to help guide my actions in the future. This might be particularly useful when I reach the stage of supporting others who are less experienced than me. Writing this reflection for my e-portfolio will mean there is an artefact that can be retrieved easily in the months and years to come: whenever it becomes relevant.

We no longer need to untangle the learning for this practitioner. S/he has displayed competence in *reflection* on important aspects of professional practice.

Reflection

Reflection is another active process that supports learning. The idea of reflection can be unpopular with students and practitioners. This is partly because attaining a useful amount of insight from reflection on episodes in the workplace or elsewhere is a skill that takes time and effort to develop. We may not really feel the benefits of reflection until we become reasonably skilful. More than this, until we become skilful it can be embarrassing to be asked to make our reflections public in, for example, assessed work or group discussions. Some senior educators argue about whether these practices destroy the value of reflection, causing people to retreat to the safety of simply describing episodes and making superficial comments about learning.

In reflection the aim is to examine what has been learnt in a way that is personally meaningful and helps to guide future actions. Ways to do this include:

- Creating recognition of a need to practise certain skills and suggesting which parts of the performance need improving
- Identifying elements of skilled performance in others that you would wish to emulate
- Identifying knowledge deficits that can then be prioritized and addressed
- Recognizing emotions stirred (in yourself or others) and deciding whether a change in your approach might be beneficial.

There will never be time to reflect on everything you do. Just think how very draining this would be! However, completely unreflective practice is likely to result in someone repeating the same behaviours and decisions over and over – probably not celebrating and building on strengths and probably not addressing weaknesses that will one day trip them up. Ultimately, professional life without reflection and development is not satisfying, so most practitioners develop some way to draw learning from the past and present to incorporate in their future actions and decisions. This helps us to learn about, from and with others.

Pause Point 5.1: Reflection

Take a moment to review Scene 5 where the practitioner is reflecting on all that's happened since s/he had the 'good idea' that physiotherapy would help the patient.

How has reflection been used as a learning tool?
What has reflection contributed to the practitioner's knowledge about their interprofessional practice?
How might all of this apply to you and your learning, and your practice?

Referral as a key part of interprofessional collaboration

In Case Study 5.1, the novice practitioner's assessment that her client could be helped by a physiotherapist begins the chain of events in the scenes that follow. This process, usually called referral, is a key aspect of professional practice; it necessitates and provides opportunities for learning from, with and about others.

Virtually every practitioner has significant elements of their workload determined by referrals from or to other practitioners or services. These may be requests to take over the care of a certain client or patient. More likely they are requests for assessment, tests, appropriate interventions and /or giving treatment; they may require giving feedback to the practitioner making the original referral or request. Responses to referrals form an important part of effective interprofessional collaboration to provide user-focused services.

In this way, the quality of referrals and the quality of responses to referrals play a large role in the quality of services. Inaccurate referrals waste resources and cause delays during which time the client's situation may deteriorate and their needs increase. These include:

- Referrals to the wrong type of practitioner or service
- Between organizations that do not have a contract or other mechanism enabling them to provide services to one another
- Referrals containing inaccurate or insufficient information.

Similarly, providing slow, incomplete or inaccurate responses to referrals wastes resources and causes delays. Many high-profile failures in care involved crucial errors in referral, such as:

- Not referring on for specialist assessment and care quickly enough
- Choosing the wrong practitioner or service for the referral
- Not providing sufficient information for others to act upon
- Not receiving information and not acting appropriately.

We return to these issues in chapter 9, which focuses on information sharing.

Referrals may be within your own profession or service, perhaps to a more experienced or specialist practitioner. These will not always feel like formal referrals, often not requiring a letter or form. Sometimes you will simply ask a colleague to make a brief assessment and advise you. Sometimes you will *hand over* a client or patient to a more experienced colleague. Nevertheless all types of referral for additional input, and the responses received, should be logged in case notes. A high proportion of referrals will be interprofessional, inter-agency or inter-service to people whom you believe possess relevant skills, knowledge and resources to progress the care of your client or patient. They may be to colleagues working in statutory services, or in voluntary and community organizations, or, increasingly, in agencies run by the private sector.

Referral can be a straightforward request from you to one other colleague; it may involve more than one person or organization. For example, if you work with people with enduring and complex needs, at times these may call for a network of referrals requiring careful coordination and sensitivity to the different ways of working of a number of colleagues. Organizing the discharge of an elderly person from an acute care ward into a nursing home is another example of a case where referral to a number of colleagues becomes necessary so that, in collaboration with the patient, their family and friends, the best possible place is found. In this situation, it is likely you will be referring your patient to colleagues in rehabilitation services and social service agencies; it is also likely that the nursing homes suitable for your patient will be in the private sector.

To select the correct people you will need to synthesize your assessment of your client's or patient's needs with knowledge about who is best placed to meet these. This is where learning about the practice of colleagues from other areas of work is valuable. It enables you to make efficient and correct referrals.

Most interprofessional, inter-agency or inter-service referrals will require the completion of a form (increasingly, an electronic form). This will at least give structure to the information you provide. It helps you to frame your request accurately and in sufficient detail to elicit a timely and accurate response. However, many referrals require significant elements of free text (sometimes a letter rather than text boxes within a form). It will be necessary to draw upon greater levels of professional knowledge, expertise and judgement to complete these. Relevant professional knowledge includes knowledge about your client or patient and about the practitioner or service that is the target of your referral; and also about rules governing the exchange of information. Expertise lies in being able to identify what is significant and communicating this effectively to the correct people. Professional judgement, acquired through synthesizing professional knowledge, expertise and reflection upon experience, guides the type and urgency of referrals made; and the urgency of following up responses to referrals. Learner Exercise 5.3 puts the spotlight on the referrals that you might make in your area of practice and where referrals might come from to you. You can do the exercise alone but it will be more enlightening if your work is shared with others, particularly if shared with people from other specialities or services. If you have the opportunity to work in an interprofessional team on the exercise, take time to compare your responses. Reflect on any differences that arose in who knew what, and consider what learning all of you might now undertake to enhance your future referral practice.

Learning Exercise 5.3: A spotlight on referrals

Think about your area of professional practice.

- To which type of practitioner or service are you likely to make referrals?
- Do you know enough about these practitioners and services to be confident that these are the most appropriate destinations for your referrals? How might you find out more? For each type of practitioner or service, do you know enough about what information can and should be included in your referral? And how best to organize and express things to help make your questions, concerns and requests as easily understood as possible? What about the varying context-specific use of technical terms and abbreviations? How might you find out more?
- From which type of practitioner or service are you likely to receive referrals? What sort of information do you need from them and how would you like that presented?
- Do you have knowledge of recurrent gaps, overlaps or confusions in information supplied in referrals? How might you work towards improving the quality of referrals received?

Other opportunities to learn about, from and with others

There are many opportunities to extend your knowledge and improve your professional practice by learning about, from and with other practitioners. These include formal education or continuing professional development (CPD) which is shared with practitioners from other professions or services. Sometimes this is overtly labelled as interprofessional education or inter-agency training. At other times, perhaps a training day on a service improvement initiative, the interprofessional aspect may not become obvious until everyone introduces themselves to each other.

Informal education or CPD is equally important and can provide valuable opportunities for interprofessional learning. It usually occurs as a by-product of other activities, and Box 5.2 has examples of these: do add in others that you know about.

Box 5.2: Opportunities for informal interprofessional learning

Audits of services, outcomes, incidents or complaints.
Processes for developing new services to meet changing needs.
Participation in the implementation of national or local quality-improvement priorities; for example:

- Reducing inappropriate hospital admissions
- Providing better end-of-life care for all
- Responding better to domestic violence incidents.

Another important opportunity for learning about, from and with others is provided by participation in team meetings of various types. Interprofessional and inter-agency meetings convened to discuss particular clients or particular working processes are excellent learning opportunities and well worth observing in advance of being expected to contribute. Case Study 5.2 explores this a little by returning to the novice practitioner we first met in Case Study 5.1. S/he is now slightly more experienced and continuing to analyse (or reflect upon) experiences to ensure that learning and learning opportunities are noticed and used. This multifaceted scenario illustrates an increasing confidence in learning about, from and with other practitioners, and shows that the lessons about preparing, thinking and consulting before acting have been learnt.

Once again we have used the device of 'scenes'. These capture key elements of learning from a longitudinal strand of professional practice that would have been conducted alongside other aspects of daily practice. These include seeing clients or patients and their families, maintaining good records, answering enquiries, making referrals, keeping up with the evidence base for professional practice and changes to policies and procedures, developing skills and supporting colleagues. Because our central character is now more effective at analysing experiences and identifying learning, there is less need for us to draw this out.

Case Study 5.2: (Pro)active learning from, about and with others

Scene 1

I've agreed to represent my profession and my employer in an *inter-agency* and *interprofessional* meeting to review and update care plans with a client who has complex needs. This time I recognized several learning needs to support advance preparation for this meeting. Some may seem rather mundane but they are important:

- Finding out how to get to the unfamiliar venue
- Finding out what I will be expected to take with me and making sure I have everything I need; and that I understand its content sufficiently well to answer questions, or know when I cannot answer questions
- Checking with more experienced colleagues how these meetings are usually run and the type of input that is usually expected
- Finding out whether any members of my immediate team attended earlier reviews and whether they can alert me to any issues to which I should be especially attentive.

After the self-inflicted embarrassment described in Case Study 5.1, feeling adequately prepared for new situations has become an important priority for this practitioner. Sometimes this leads to over-preparation to compensate for limited confidence. With more experience, the practitioner will find a successful balance between entering situations inadequately prepared and striving too hard for comprehensive preparation, given the reality that professional encounters are intrinsically unpredictable and time is always in short supply.

Case Study 5.2 continued

Scene 2

Attending the multiprofessional review was quite scary but I learnt so much, for example:

- Suddenly I became acutely aware that I was there to represent the views of my profession and the views of the service where I work, not just my own thoughts – although I was expected to have thoughts of my own. Sometimes it felt as if these multiple perspectives only partly overlapped, with some aspects of them seeming to conflict. Did I need to develop multiple personalities?
- Some of the things I thought were really important were hardly mentioned by other people. I wasn't sure how much I could or should press my points. I must remember to talk to my supervisor about this.
- At certain moments it felt as if everyone present had a different priority and we were not going to get anywhere. The review meeting chair was quite skilful:

she kept reminding us of the priorities the client had described. Gradually people began to rephrase what they thought was important to include, mentioning how this linked to one or more things from the client's priorities. Once people began to describe their priorities in this way many things seemed more reasonable and obvious. People began to identify what they could usefully contribute and a sensible sequence for things to happen; they also began to say how long they thought certain things would take and how soon they thought progress should be reviewed.

- I was pleased that I managed to make two well-received suggestions – I must do the follow-up work relating to these. For the rest of the time I tried to listen hard and observe people's behaviour. That way, while I was learning about this particular case I was also learning things that will be useful for clients with similar needs; and I was learning how these important meetings work.

- Listening to people, particularly when they were rephrasing their advice in the light of the client's priorities, I realized that certain words and phrases have slightly different meanings for different professions or different services. That created some confusion when everyone was stating their initial priorities. It also seemed as if there could be multiple names for the same thing. I will have to try to remember as many variations as possible and check more carefully that I really understand what has been asked of me.

In scene 2 we see a good balance between focusing on yourself, the processes in the social interaction, the needs of the client and family, and the behaviour of others. These elements include your own feelings, your contributions to the shared discussion and your learning needs; language and ways of thinking leading to misunderstandings or conflicting priorities; strategies to overcome misunderstanding and conflict; observation of strengths worth emulating and weaknesses to try to avoid.

Case Study 5.2 continued

Scene 3

At one point, the work of the case conference came to a standstill because important results from a regional assessment unit were not available. This will delay things for the client, which nobody wants. It also means that quite a few people here today will have to reconvene when the results come through, which is inefficient. Nobody was sure who had been expected to check the results were available, chasing up if necessary. Nobody was volunteering today either! The chair cut short the beginning of a debate on this incident as another example of poor communication between the regional centre and local services, but she would not move on until one person had agreed to follow up the results for this particular client. I was impressed.

Actively noticing what is happening when something impresses us is an important part of learning about, from and with other practitioners. In this case an experienced meeting chair was preventing unproductive descent into blaming, as well as ensuring that everyone knew the proposed way forward from the impasse. We shall see in a moment that outside the meeting she followed up by starting attempts to address the underlying system-failure. Attention to systemic problems is normally more productive than spotlighting the perceived failings of individuals, although of course serious or persistent weakness in individual performance cannot be ignored.

Case Study 5.2 continued

Scene 4

After the inter-agency interprofessional case review I had some follow-up work to complete. It went well and I feel much more confident about my next big case review. We also received an email from the review chair saying that she wanted to convene a small group that would look at the systems in place to ensure that all relevant results will be available for complex case reviews. I think this is important work that could make a real difference for clients and everyone who works with them – although I wonder if we will notice: people tend to notice when things go wrong and take the same things for granted when they are working well. It is not appropriate for me to join this small systems-improvement group. At the moment I have more than enough to do in learning the basic job; and I am not sure that I yet have the organizational knowledge and authority to contribute effectively.

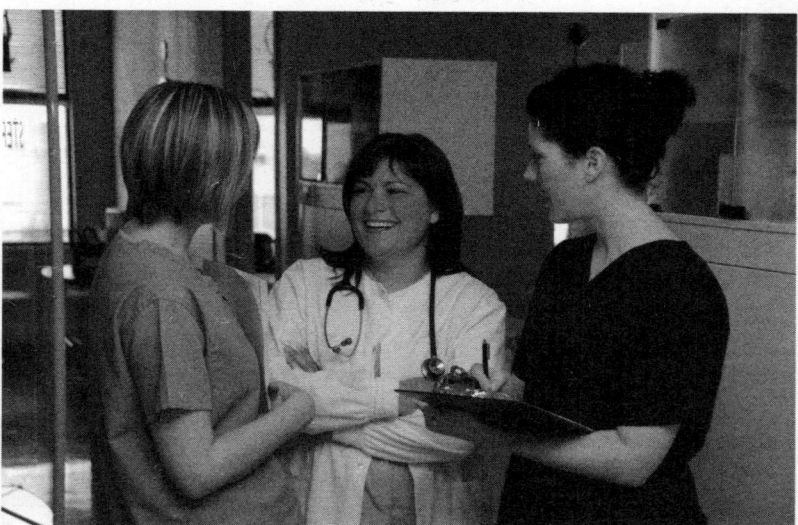

Photo 5.4 Never be afraid to ask! There is so much that can be learnt from colleagues both within and outside your own profession. Vicki Reid/iStock.

In our final scene the novice practitioner is making well-received profession-specific contributions within the currently attained level of professional expertise, as well as making good decisions about when it is not appropriate to respond to a request for assistance.

To conclude

Both the scenarios used in this chapter show how *problems*, gaps between what we know and what we feel we need to know, or gaps between what is happening and what we would like to happen, stimulate learning. But it's important to remember that learning is also stimulated by a human or professional desire continually to do things better. In other words, we take a critical look at our current performance and label some aspects of this as *problems* which we wish to address through active learning.

During professional practice, *problems* of various types and degrees of complexity punctuate our working days. Some fit a pattern that we recognize and we may be able to implement a tried and tested response. Otherwise, some deeper engagement and original thinking will be required.

Away from daily practice, meaningful active learning may be encouraged by professional education and CPD that is case-based (real cases or vignettes designed to draw out key points) and through problem-based and enquiry-based learning (PBL, EBL), through engagement with simulation. You can also use individual learning plans developed with reference to the reality of your practice. All these tools will help you to learn to work better both independently and collaboratively.

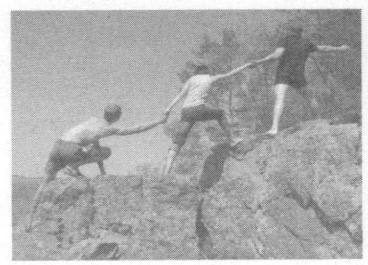

Learning About, From and With Service Users

You must be the change you wish to see in the world.

Mahatma Gandhi

What you will read in this chapter

Earlier chapters of this book have indicated being an interprofessional practitioner is not only about learning and working with others in the workforce; it is also about learning and working with the people who use the services you deliver. For example, in chapter 2 we used a publication for young learning-disabled adults, written in consultation with young learning-disabled adults, as an example of being interprofessional arising from personal development initiatives.

In other words, we are arguing that the work you do is done with people who use your services, and not to them. In this case, the word 'people' means children, young people and adults. Everyone involved in this way of working learns about, from and with each other, as needs are assessed and the delivery of services are planned.

In this chapter we look at why working with people who use services is important, and at some policies that support this collaborative way of working. We show some of the ways of making this sometimes difficult way of working successful. You will read about examples to illustrate how everyone can learn about, from and with each other – the client you support, the person you care for, the child or young person you teach, and practitioners in the interprofessional team. Some different aspects of learning and working with users of services are detailed. These include the story of a young boy, Timothy, his illness and his life, and comments on how service users made a difference to a research project. As in previous chapters, there are learner exercises and pause points to encourage you to apply what we write about in your work setting.

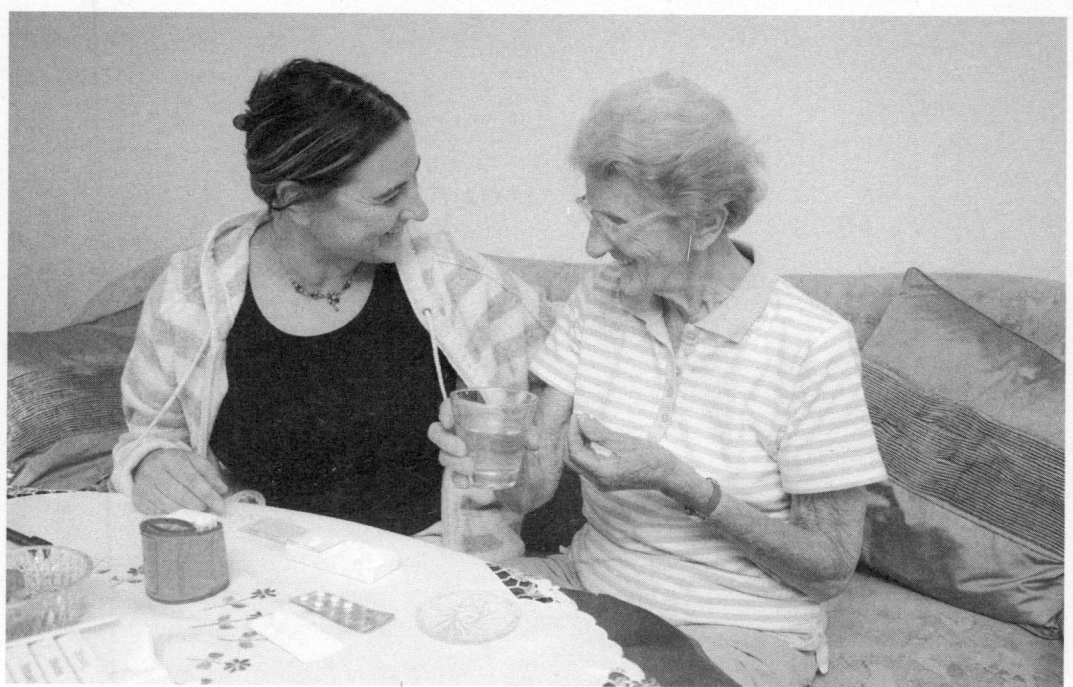

Photo 6.1 Listening to service users and learning from them is a central foundation of good interprofessional practice. Annett Vauteck/iStock.

Learning and working together

To highlight the distinctiveness of learning and working with service users as an equal part of the interprofessional team, we refer to this as learning and working together. In other books or papers you will find it referred to as learning for partnership or collaborative work.

In the next chapter we focus on unpaid carers as equally important in the learning and working team. This separation highlights that the service user and their unpaid carer are distinctive and different. However, because of the close relationship between users and their carers, there are places in this chapter where carers are also referred to. In this chapter our aim is to focus on what it means to think of users as an integral part of the interprofessional team in both an education and practice context. Our emphasis is on the learning and working together, whether this is during a formal education course or during your working life. We see this as a two-way process which continues throughout your career as a practitioner. Interprofessional training and practice often focuses on how to work interprofessionally with practitioners from other disciplines. Viewing service users themselves as an integral part of the interprofessional team, with their own voice and viewpoints, is equally important and has its own history and characteristics. The aim is that public services should be delivered in ways much more in tune with the needs of people receiving them.

How did the move for service-user involvement in public services come about? User involvement in practice and training emerged from changes in thinking about public services. In the UK, two diverse currents of thought informed these changes. The first was a set of ideas in the 1960s and 1970s which challenged established practices and the power of practitioners and authorities to make decisions on behalf of others. This approach emphasized social justice, social inclusion (see chapter 8) and community development approaches, and was linked to the new social movements, such as feminism, the movements for race equality and disability rights. It focused on the structural inequalities in society and the way in which certain groups of people, for instance those with learning disabilities (as shown later in Timothy's story), were often stigmatized, marginalized and excluded.

The second set of ideas that gained ground in the 1980s and 1990s came from a different current of thought. In this, the focus was on breaking up the monolithic power of public services, and shifting power from practitioners to the user as a *customer* with choices. It argued that there were lessons for the public services in the way that the private sector was organized and managed. This approach is sometimes called the *supermarket* model (Winkler 1994) or new managerialism. In the UK, both these shifts in thought resulted in a government desire for public services to be more person-led. The move to direct payments to service users to purchase their own care is a result of this drive.

The changes were driven by the view that this would contribute to improvements not only in the service users' experience, but also in service quality and the value for money of that service (DoH 2006, p. 16). As such, it was thought to be a more popular and acceptable approach than the rather autocratic systems it sought to replace. The first quote below shows how this was talked about at the time by the prime minster's office. It was then translated into policy statements, as the examples from UK government departments in the following quotes show. To read more about these policies, use the websites at the end of the quotes. In the following section, we look at the evolution of these statements of policies for service-user participation in public services at the beginning of the twenty-first century.

We are proposing to put an entirely different dynamic in place to drive our public services: one where the service will be driven not by the managers but by the user. (Prime Minister, the Rt Hon. Tony Blair MP, July 2004) <http://archive.cabinetoffice.gov.uk/opsr/documents/rtf/leafletng.rtf> (accessed 9 September 2008)

. . . the learner is a partner in learning, not a passive recipient – and this means that (especially as they grow older, leaving compulsory education),they have a stake in and a responsibility for their own learning, *and* (with the state) moving away from (setting the) direction towards an enabling and empowering role. (UK Secretary of State for Educations and Skills 2004) <http://www.dfes.gov.uk/publications/5yearstrategy/> (accessed 9 September 2008)

The involvement of patients, carers and the public in health decision-making is at the heart of the modernisation of the NHS. (Department of Health and Farrell 2004)

. . . recognition of the skills of patients and carers in managing chronic conditions. (Department of Health and Farrell 2004; <http://www.dh.gov.uk/en/Publicationsandstatistics/ Publications/PublicationsPolicyAndGuidance/DH_4082332> (accessed 9 September 2008)

We want to give individuals and their friends and families greater control over the way in which social care supports their needs. (Green Paper: *Independence, Well-being and Choice: Our Vision for the Future of Social Care for Adults in England*; available at: <http://www.dh.gov.uk/en/Publicationsandstatistics/ Publications/PublicationsPolicyAndGuidance/DH_4106477>; accessed 9 September 2008).

And:

We want to provide better information and signposting to allow people to retain responsibility, and to put people at the centre of assessing their own needs and how those needs can best be met. (Green Paper: *Independence, Well-being and Choice: Our Vision for the Future of Social Care for Adults in England*) <http://www.dh.gov.uk/en/Publicationsandstatistics/ Publications/PublicationsPolicyAndGuidance/DH_4106477> (accessed 9 September 2008)

Policies for participation

In Figure 6.1 we suggest a way of looking at the development of user-focused services from a European and UK human rights legislation perspective. Ideally, policies for these services then translate into practices that deliver enhanced services focused on the needs of the individual service user. The model begins and ends with human rights for all, which aims to support the practice of equal access to services for all, equal treatment within them, and practices which challenge discrimination against individual service users. A human rights approach supports the recognition of everyone's right to participate in decisions about their own life and the lives of those they help and care for. For example, in health and social care settings, the policies required:

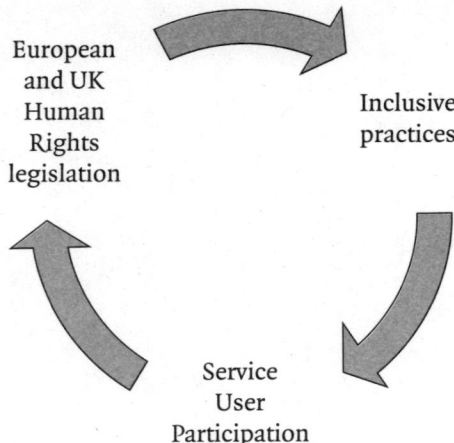

European
and UK
Human
Rights
legislation

Inclusive
practices

Service
User
Participation

Figure 6.1 An ideological framework for the development of service-user participation

More choice and a strong voice for patients and service users who will be able, in consultation with their clinicians, to choose the highest quality of care appropriate for their needs. (DoH 2006, p. 10)

And in children's services policy-makers said that:

We want to see services delivered around the needs of the child, not around the specialism of a particular practitioner or agency. Increasingly this will involve practitioners working in a multi-agency setting, where they are part of an integrated children's service rather than an individual service for children. (DfES, 2007, p. 21)

So one way of looking at why service users should be part of the interprofessional learning team is by seeing this as promoting human rights with equal rights for all citizens. In other words, recognizing a common humanity and treating people accordingly.

To take one example, historically people with disabilities have been discriminated against. They were often put in institutions and segregated from other people in society. They were seen as *different* and without the right to make decisions about their own lives. The Disability Discrimination Act(s) (1995, 2005) (DDA) seek to challenge that and to ensure that people with disabilities receive equal treatment.

Discrimination can be hard to see. An example of less visible discrimination is that people with a history of mental health problems still find it hard to get jobs, even in the health services. Although the DDA give a certain amount of protection to disabled people, including people with some mental health conditions, discrimination can be hard to pinpoint and prove. Difficult interprofessional dilemmas can arise where there are competing human rights issues.

Pause Point 6.1: Reflection on discrimination

Have a look at the Disability Discrimination Act (1995 and 2005). A good place to start looking at this is <www.directgov.co.uk> – the government website.

Who is the Act seeking to protect?
Who is defined as disabled under the Act?
How do the Acts seek to make sure that disabled people are included in:

- Health and social care services?
- Education?

What barriers are there to inclusion in your setting? Think not only about physical access to buildings but, for example, the availability of staff who can sign for deaf people?
    What other forms of accessibility need to be considered?
    Now look at the website for People First: <www.peoplefirstld.com>. How is disability viewed by this organization of people with learning disabilities?

Some women with learning disabilities still have their children taken into care. This may happen if the specialist services which might help to support them in looking after their children are not easily accessible. There are also examples of good practice, where experience of using the mental health system or having a disability is seen as an advantage for an employee, a service user or a member of the interprofessional team. At the end of this chapter, Sheryl talks about her experiences of being involved in a mental health project where the experience of being a service user was valued.

Legislation and policy about equal opportunities have had an impact on all aspects of our personal and working lives. The Human Rights Act (1998), the Sex Discrimination Act (1975), the Race Relations Act (1976), the Disability Discrimination Act (1995), and the Equal Treatment Regulations from Europe (2007), made discrimination against gay men and lesbians illegal. This affects us all as employees, employers or as people delivering services in an interprofessional context.

The rules and guidelines on these subjects provide a foundation for how we relate to others, what we ourselves expect from others, and how organizations and institutions behave towards their staff and the public they serve. They have in common a principle of inclusion and of the right to have a say in the choices made about what happens to you.

The policy and practice of user involvement and the promotion of user participation in public service provision use this ideology of inclusion. We devised Learner Exercise 6.1 so that you can relate the general and political policies to the realities of your practice. The exercise aims to help you understand more about the complexity of

Learner Exercise 6.1: The influence of policy on my practice

1 Make some notes of how one of the policies in the quotes on p. 108 relates to your professional practice setting. You can read more about the policy on the websites indicated.
2 What organizations and agencies would be involved in delivering the services related to that policy to service users?
3 How many members of the workforce team from these organizations and agencies would be involved in implementing the policy you chose?
4 Draw a connections map of how these people might interact with each other and the user of the service they are providing. A connections map uses different colours and line types to give a picture of interactions between people. For example, you can use thick lines to indicate strong connections, broken lines for weak connections, and wavy or crossed lines where there is stress associated with the connection.

user participation and the potential for one or more of a service user's needs (be they a pupil, client or patient) to be overlooked.

Government statements with admirable aims are easily made and you will probably be able to find many more, because writing the aims is possibly the easiest part of the process. However, delivering person-focused services has resource implications, and critics have wondered if the policies are able to live up to their promises in the context of limited budgets and the marketization of care (Pollock 2004). The next step is to ensure that policies for person-focused services make a differences to the service user. In Pause Point 6.2 we've started to list some of the issues involved when it comes to translating policy into practice. You could see how these apply to the policy for person-focused services in your field of practice. Either think about these issues by yourself or, ideally, do this with learners from other professions *and* with some service users.

Please remember to first ask their permission to learn with them in this way. As a student, you are probably very familiar with exchanging your opinions with others – after all, that's one way of learning. If you do this with service users who participate in the teaching on your course this way of learning may be unfamiliar to them. It might feel rather intimidating, so introduce what you want to do with this in mind and be prepared to stop if necessary. Remember that thinking and talking about these issues is likely to bring in your own and others' politics, and to highlight how it feels being on the receiving end of service delivery.

By now you will have realized that putting policies into practice depends on the service involved. It also depends on who has written the policy because these come not only from government departments, but also from service organizations like local authorities

Pause Point 6.2: Policies into practice

The policy aim that services should be person-led might not make a difference in practice or, if a difference is made, it might not be the one that everyone hoped for because:

- Policies change when they become reality
- Not everyone translates the policy in the same way
- The policy was written without knowing enough about its delivery context
- The people writing the policy had a hidden agenda.

Can you add to this list?

and health-care trusts. One of the issues you might have become aware of when reading Pause Point 6.2 is that many organizational policies ripple out from central or local government policies. Even individual departments are likely to have their own policies: it's a good idea to ask to see these if you are on a placement. They translate the wider policy for the local context and it can be easier to see what this type of policy means for staff.

Returning to more general policies, we now look at the ways different publicly funded services show how they are putting the government's directives for person-focused services into practice. For this, we set ourselves the relatively easy task of an Internet search, limited to UK sites and two areas of public service, to see different ways in which the views of service users were being heard and used. We were particularly interested in initiatives that could be easily found and adapted for local use; to us, this means efficient and more effective use of resources. In turn we report our findings for:

- Children's services; and
- Health-care services.

Children's participation and children's services

Our examples here focus on work being done through the Every Child Matters agenda. We found information on: <http://www.everychildmatters.gov.uk/participation/faq> (accessed 6 January 2008) about young people's ideas of how best to listen to what they say about services for them (Box 6.1).

There is a lot more about this on the Every Child Matters website, including a pdf document, *Learning to Listen: Core Principles for the Involvement of Children and Young People*. If you are particularly interested in work that involves children and young people, then it's worthwhile downloading this from: <http://www.everychildmatters.gov.uk/_files /1F85704C1D67D71E30186FEBCEDED6D6.pdf> (accessed 6 January 2008). It looks at what participation is and its importance, and has case studies and examples to show how participation can work.

Box 6.1: What do young people say about participation and how it can be done effectively?

- It won't happen without the right resources to support it
- Make sure there is flexibility about meeting times so they can happen at times that suit young people
- Staff with the right skills need to be specifically dedicated to support young people's participation; make sure there are enough staff to make a difference
- Make sure a range of methods is used for communicating with young people in ways they will find easy, such as text messaging
- Make sure we give good feedback to young people about how they have contributed
- Make sure we provide clear, ongoing communication about how the participation process will develop and what concrete action has been taken
- Always provide clear, relevant information
- Organizations should always be prepared to take feedback about themselves from young people
- Decision-makers need to get to know young people they are working with: make sure they actually meet them and show they value them
- Make sure we get the atmosphere right and use methods and approaches that don't exclude particular groups of young people
- Make sure we are always culturally inclusive
- Make sure this is enjoyable for all concerned.

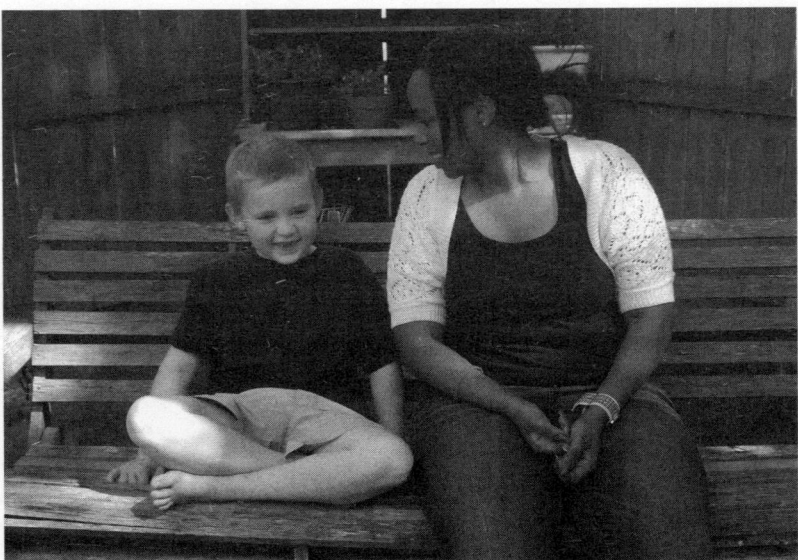

Photo 6.2 Every Child Matters has enabled young people's voices to be heard: this means young people have been able to give plenty of information on how those who work with children could improve their practice; how might you need to amend your practice if you were working with a child? Jamie Wilson/iStock.

Patient/user participation – some examples from health and social care

Since the late 1980s there has been a growth in the number and scope of programmes aiming to involve users and carers actively in the planning, delivery and evaluation of health and social care. At an individual level community care legislation has given adult service users the right to involvement in constructing their own care, with support packages that provide choice and greater flexibility to the user. At an organizational level, a range of initiatives have sought to give patients, users and carers a greater say in services which were traditionally dominated by practitioners.

The following paragraphs give a brief summary of some of these initiatives, mainly drawn from health settings. We have chosen these health examples as they illustrate a shift within a profession that has a strong hierarchical tradition and many of us will experience health care at some point in our lives. These examples are intended to show ways in which the drive for more patient- and user/carer-focused care is being taken forward. Do remember that projects move on. If some of the websites are no longer available at the time of your reading, try to find other similar work and look at what has made it successful.

Expert patient programmes

People in developed countries live longer than ever before and many patients, especially those with long-term or chronic conditions, often understand more about their conditions than anyone else. Expert patient programmes were set up by the UK Department of Health, recognizing that people with long-term conditions such as arthritis, diabetes, strokes and cancers are often expert in their own care. It is worthwhile finding out more about how this programme is progressing in your area of learning and work. One way is via: <http://www.bbc.co.uk/radio4/science/expertpatient.shtml> (accessed 8 January 2008), where you can listen to a 2005 investigation about the expert patient programme and download the programme transcript.

Students and practitioners can benefit from the experience and expertise of patients like Emma Wicks, who is the expert patient adviser at the UK Cystic Fibrosis Trust. An article about her experience can be downloaded from: <http://www.bmj.com/cgi/content/full/334/7606/0> (accessed 9 September 2008). Emma writes about her experiences of living with cystic fibrosis, in the British Medical Journal (Wicks 2007). An interprofessional team is likely to be working with Emma and her parents as she makes the transition from paediatric care to adult care. Each member of that team has something to learn from reading what Emma thinks about transition: learning that can help them to be interprofessional.

DIPEx – How do patients experience health and illness?

DIPEx (<www.dipex.org>) was set up as a resource for patients, carers, family and friends, doctors, nurses and other health practitioners in 2001, and as a training tool. Two doctors established the site after their own experience of illness, one with breast cancer and the other having had knee replacement surgery. Although they both knew the relevant medical information, they could not find anyone else to talk with about what it was really like to have their illness/condition. The website contains interviews with everyday people talking about their own experiences of serious illness and different health problems. It provides reliable information about each illness. The aim is to cover 100 conditions eventually and, by providing patients with good-quality information, to ensure they have the knowledge and power to take part in decision-making with health-care practitioners. Have a look at this resource to see if it can be of use in your work.

Involving patients and the public in health – does it work?

Evidence from twelve research projects that focused on the involvement of patients and the public in health can be downloaded from: <http://www.dh.gov.uk/en/Publicationsandstatistics/Publications/PublicationsPolicyAndGuidance/DH_4082332> (accessed 9 September 2008). This UK government-funded report, *Patient and Public Involvement: The Evidence for Policy Implementation* (DoH and Farrell 2004), provides useful information about how patients and the public feel and act when becoming involved in health provision. The report has some useful sections. In particular, there are suggestions for enhancing communication between practitioners and patients (p. 42). If you belong to an interprofessional learning group that includes service users, then agreeing a group list of good communication practices based on suggestions in this document would be a good start to your work together.

Supporting involvement

The NHS Centre for Involvement is a UK Department of Health funded body that supports public and patient involvement in health-care provision. It seeks to influence and support programmes that involve patients and the public in health policy and decision-making (see Box 6.2). Note that the list includes service users, carers and the workforce.

Lay appointments to professional bodies

There has been an increasing interest from professional bodies in widening their knowledge base through the inclusion of lay members

---

Box 6.2: Some of the work of the NHS Involvement Centre

Patient and public involvement is part of everyone's role in the NHS. Therefore, all staff need the competencies (skills, knowledge and capabilities) for involvement and diversity. The Learning and Support Domain embraces the following key elements in order to achieve this vision:

Future workforce – ensuring that all commissioned health care education and training programmes are 'patient focused' involving service users at every level; in the commissioning, design, delivery and review. Alongside this is the need to ensure that the future workforce is competent at the point of qualification to undertake those involvement activities that are commensurate with their role.

Current workforce – ensuring that all staff are clear about what expectations there are about their level of competence in involvement activities and supporting their learning and development needs.

Service Users and Carers – as the level of public involvement grows so does the need for personal training and development opportunities for patients and the wider public.

(<http://www.nhscentreforinvolvement.nhs.uk/index.cfm?content=79&Menu=29>; accessed 8 January 2008)

---

who have experienced their services. Most social work organizations from the General Social Care Council to local authority social work departments have users and carers as board members and advisers. The Social Care Institute for Excellence has looked at the impact of service user participation in social care services (Carr 2004). You can download their findings from: <www.scie.org.uk>.

The Patient and Carer Network, which advises the Royal College of Physicians, is an example of this trend in health services. It is described at <http://www.rcplondon.ac.uk/college/PIU/piu_pcn.asp> (accessed 8 January 2008). Appointments to this network are organized by the medical professional body and advertised in a variety of ways. Someone applying to join it is treated rather like someone applying for a job. Candidates submit information about themselves and references are sought. While it is important for professional bodies to take account of patient and carer views, successful applicants could feel it is similar to taking an unpaid job.

Although welcomed by patients and user/carer organizations, the involvement of lay voices in professional bodies also presents some dilemmas. Patients, ex-patients, users and carers might wish to take part but not have the time and resources. They might find the kind of language used at meetings unfamiliar or feel that their views do not carry weight. One dilemma for users or carers is that to become an effective lay adviser often requires the confidence to put across a different point of view, as well as knowledge about how to influence an organization. This is more easily gained by ongoing involvement. But staying close to the experience of other users or carers, being able to reflect their difficulties and not becoming 'professionalized' or distant from the experiences can be a challenge. Professional bodies often have considerable power and influence. The principle of appointing users and carers to DOH working groups, medical committees and social care organizations has generally been welcomed. Making the most of this input, in terms of improving service delivery, requires skilful people who know how to learn about, from and with each other.

Involving service users and carers in social work education

United Kingdom social work university education departments now have to involve users and carers in their activities, including student admissions, delivering programmes and assessing students. Nottingham University has service users and carers planning, delivering and assessing students in one of their modules called Advocacy in Action. The module raises issues about the power dynamics of communication with service users. Students give a presentation of their life history bearing in mind the communication skills they use. Some assessors may have learning or other disabilities. The students talk about what brought them to social work and are graded by the service user/carer assessors on their communication skills (Levin 2004). Are service users involved in your education programme? If so, how has user and carer involvement in your training influenced your practice? If not, what could they contribute to your learning?

To summarize so far

This chapter has looked at the reasons for learning and working with service users, highlighting some of the policies that aim to put this into practice. You will also have read about ways in which service users participate in making sure these practices are authentic and reflect the reality of their lives. Much of what we've written has been general so now we move on to look at how this is put into practice.

Timothy's story

In this section we focus on understanding some practical ways in which service users can be as much a part of the interprofessional learning team as those involved in delivering services are. We do this through the example of **Timothy's** story (pp. 117–18). In other chapters you will find examples of how different members of the workforce form the team that delivers a service to a person. What they all have in common is the potential for the practitioners to learn not only about, from, and with each other, but also and importantly, for practitioners to learn about from, and with the service user and their carer.

You will have met similar situations in your specific area of practice. In some teams you will be making a large contribution to the service delivered, while in other teams your expertise may be needed once in a while, and sometimes you may have a small and very passing role. What will remain the same is the person who needs care and support; they are always there. They hold the collective memory of their needs and the ways in which these have or have not been met. Their knowledge is unique and irreplaceable.

In a collaborative practice team, it is likely that different members of it will use different words to describe the person at the centre of the team. They will, of course, provide different services to Timothy and his family. The story of Timothy illustrates this and some of the other issues that arise when a young child becomes seriously ill with a chronic condition. Learner Exercise 6.2 is designed to help you understand more about:

- Differences in language within the interprofessional team
- Ways in which Timothy's team see their part in looking after him.

You can do Learner Exercise 6.2 by yourself, but as it concerns how the interprofessional team collaborates with Timothy and his parents to ensure all his learning and care needs are met, it would be good to work with students from other professions.

Case Study 6.1: Timothy's story

The vitamin that may give Timothy his childhood back

A ten-year-old boy paralysed by a condition so rare that it has been named after him is slowly starting to recover, thanks to a doctor's hunch.

Timothy Bingham was two years old when a flu-like illness left him temporarily unable to walk. Three years later he lost control of his body and since then has been confined to a wheelchair, able to communicate only by eye movement.

His condition baffled doctors for years and it was only when a specialist in metabolic diseases suspected he might be lacking a vital amino acid that his condition began to improve.

The missing amino acid, which helps muscles to communicate, is called L-serine and Timothy has been taking it three times a day since October. Now he can hold his head up, wiggle his toes and talk. 'I couldn't do a lot of stuff that I can now. I feel positive about the future,' he said yesterday.

His parents, Kate and Richard, of Cheltenham, are equally optimistic about their boy getting his life back. Mrs Bingham, a council worker, said: 'As a mother, you need to hope that there may be somebody out there one day who finds the miracle you've been searching for. I never lost hope. We don't know whether this will be a cure but we're keeping everything crossed that this is.'

Mrs Bingham and her husband, an engineer, said that after Timothy first collapsed, specialists at the Radcliffe Hospital, Oxford, told them they suspected that he was suffering from Guillain-Barre syndrome, where the body's immune system attacks part of the nervous system. After dozens of tests they could not conclusively prove the diagnosis so they named the mystery condition Bingham syndrome.

Timothy's condition improved and he returned to leading a normal life. It was not to last for long. His second collapse was the most devastating. His mother watched as his body went limp, limb by limb, and by the time he arrived at the Cheltenham General Hospital, he had stopped breathing and was put on a ventilator.

Doctors at the Radcliffe referred the couple to Professor Peter Clayton, a professor of metabolic medicine at Great Ormond Street Hospital and the Institute of Child Health, who concluded last October that vitamin deficiency could be the problem.

He worked out that Timothy produced only small amounts of L-serine and stopped completely during the periods of flu when he was eating less.

'We carried out an extensive series of tests and noticed this amino acid was rather low in his blood,' he said.

Although Professor Clayton has described Timothy's progress as 'outstanding' he said that it was too early to be certain of a total cure.

'Obviously we are delighted with Tim's progress so far. He has got a lot more movement in his arms. However, I think we need to be cautious. There has been one other case described before and that patient did benefit from serine treatment, but I think we should not assume too much at this stage.'

Mrs Bingham said: 'He lost his voice so he was trying to communicate with his eyes. His brain was intact so he couldn't understand why his body wasn't moving. He wasn't even able to blink.

'This has been like climbing a mountain every day for five years and now it feels like we're getting near to the top.

'When the attack happened, he just fell to his side . . . I still have nightmares about that moment. It was such a terrible shock because I didn't know if I was watching my son die. Our whole life was turned upside-down. We became carers overnight, which is something nobody prepares you for. He's always been an outdoorsy child, climbing trees and playing football. This vitamin might just have given us the chance to get that boy back.'

Only one case of a person suffering recurrent paralysis and recovering has been documented – a girl in Iran, who went on to make a full recovery.

The Times, 20 March 2007. Reproduced with permission

You may have noticed that in Learner Exercise 6.2 we included the work of the practitioners in Timothy's care team and asked you to look at their perspectives and how working in this way highlights differences in the language they use and their perceived importance on the team. We hope you realized what was missing from this!

So far, we haven't asked you to think about how all this appears to Timothy and his parents. Leaving their perspectives out, or until the end, is more common than it should be. Learning and working together means treating everyone in a fair and equal way.

Pause Point 6.3 redresses the balance lost by not including Timothy and his parents in Learner Exercise 6.2. It is not possible for you or anyone else to know how they feel, what they want and how they see everyone in the care team. But often it is the role of the practitioner to find out about these things. That can be a very difficult task. Ask yourself the questions in Pause Point 6.3 with the example

---

Learner Exercise 6.2: The 'who's who' of Timothy's care team

Read Timothy's story.
Make a list of everyone involved in helping Timothy in his daily life.

If you are working with colleagues, compare your lists and compile a group list from each individual list.

If you are working on your own, select two people from your list and think about who they might want added to the list.

Write a short note on how everybody on the list relates to Timothy, and include the word they would use to describe him in relation to themselves. For example, Timothy's occupational therapist might say 'one part of my work for this patient was to assess how the family bathroom needed adapting so that he could have a shower and use the toilet'. Share your notes with others and discuss any differences in the name and words used.

Now put the people on the final list in the order that you think shows their importance in:

- Enabling Timothy to live his life
- Supporting Timothy's parents.

Discuss any similarities and differences in this order between the different lists in your group. Talk about the reasons for these. If you are working on your own, re-order the people as if you were a different practitioner working with Timothy and his family. What differences are there when you do this from the perspective of different people in Timothy's interprofessional care team?

Pause Point 6.3: Service users' and carers' needs

Finding out what service users need and how they want their needs to be met takes a lot of skill and sometimes has to be done in a very short time.

- What sort of questions might give you useful answers about these needs?
- What difficulties might you meet when asking your questions?
- What else could you do to understand more about service user and carer needs?

of Timothy and his parents in mind. Make some notes about your answers; assess whether you would have been successful in finding what you needed to know. Has practising doing this as part of your studies changed how you might work with service users to complete a needs assessment for them?

Spaces for learning together

This chapter has focused on the importance of listening to what service users know about their needs and the services they want to meet their needs. This means working with them to help shape those services and recognizing that their knowledge is valuable. Increasingly, service users participate in the recruitment, teaching and assessing of students on university courses. We have touched before on ways that encourage participation, and in this section we look specifically at the importance of the environment in which formal learning happens.

One aspect of learning together that's central to how service users feel about participating is how comfortable they are in the places and spaces where learning takes place. It's important to recognize the different life experiences that members of this novel learning team may have had. There will be service users without the experience of going on to a university campus, somewhere that can seem a confusing and intimidating place to a newcomer. That's one reason why first-year undergraduate students have orientation programmes: finding out where to go for a drink, how to get to the library, and what times the bus goes between different sites.

Making sure everyone feels welcome is a good start for any collaborative working group. However, not only the place of learning but also the space can create the optimal setting for learning about, from and with each other. Entering a building full of lecture theatres with seating in rows may feel like going back to school, perhaps with bad memories of difficult times for some people. These types of buildings fitted more traditional teaching-centred models of education; they are a poor fit in an age that recognizes the importance of student-centred education, with individual learning styles and the influences of technology. This has been acknowledged by groups organizing this type of learning, so new spaces have been created that encourage participation and collaborative learning. In such a space everyone can contribute equally to learning about, from and with each other, and have their individual learning needs met.

You may be learning somewhere that feels less like a traditional university and more like a place everyone can go into for all sorts of learning experiences. One example is the new building that houses the Centre of Excellence in Interdisciplinary Mental Health (CEIMH) at the University of Birmingham, UK, a partnership between six university disciplines, key local, national and international mental health agencies, and service user and carer organizations. Box 6.3 summarizes the aims of the new building and shows the participatory nature of its creation. The CEIMH website <http://www.ceimh.bham. ac.uk/> (accessed 9 September 2008) highlights that:

> . . . service-users and carers played a major part in the design and 'feel' of the building in order to ensure an atmosphere of 'comfort' for everyone who enters it.

and

> During the design phase the staff, service-users and carers were acutely aware of and argued for the need to ensure that different teaching and learning styles were catered for.

Box 6.3: Creation of a welcoming all-together-learning space at Birmingham University, UK

The design of the Centre of Excellence in Interdisciplinary Mental Health has been influenced by a number of perspectives including input from mental health teaching and administrative staff, practitioners and service users and carers to ensure that it is:

Flexible – to accommodate current and evolving teaching and learning approaches.
Welcoming – to ensure that every perspective within the mental health field is heard and valued.
Creative – to develop the potential of learners of all ages.
Innovative – to allow access to different forms of digital expression by accommodating a multimedia production facility.
Supportive – to develop the potential for interdisciplinary activity.
Accessible – to inclusively accommodate the learning needs of a diverse range of students, practitioners, service users and carers.

It is the aim of the CEIMH to ensure that the environment provides a space that motivates learners and promotes collaborative teaching and learning activity that is personalised and inclusive. The part that technology will play is to ensure that there is a level of flexibility that meets everyone's needs.

Taken from <http://www.ceimh.bham.ac.uk/centre/location.shtml>
(accessed 10 January 2008)

Of course, much more than learning and teaching happens in a university; these institutions not only have a role in the reproduction of knowledge, but also in knowledge production through research and development work. We think it's equally important to listen to what service users know during research activities that aim to fill the gaps in our collective knowledge. Not only this; it's important to then use the new knowledge to change practices and service delivery, as well as what students learn about these. We now turn to an example of how service users became an integral part of a research project, leading to changes in practice.

Participatory research with mental health service users – user involvement in practice

The project described here sought the perspectives of mental health service users on community and hospital care (Rose 2001). One key aspect of the enquiry process was the participation of mental health service users as researchers in the data collection process. You've probably read enough research reports to know that this is quite unusual. This type of participation provides a better balance of power between the *researchers* and the *researched*. It leads to more relevant research questions, as the person answering the questions is more confident that they and their responses will be taken seriously.

The project took place over several years. During this time, sixty-one mental health service-user interviewers were trained under the auspices of the Sainsbury Centre for Mental Health. They then interviewed over 500 mental health service users living in the community and in hospitals, and from different inner-city and rural areas of England. The questions they asked were developed by the user interviewers themselves. They were involved in analysing the data collected. One of the project's findings was that the service users being interviewed relaxed and opened up once they knew that the interviewer had also been through the mental health system and understood their situation. The fact that the interviewers were service users themselves made a huge difference to the interviewees. The interviewers said that they also benefited from carrying out the interviews. They valued taking part in a group research process and learning new skills. Most importantly, their experience of having been through the mental health system became valued rather than devalued and stigmatizing.

Here is what one interviewer, Sheryl, wrote about her experiences of interviewing in Huntingdon:

> I was still in hospital when I first heard about the project.
> On a little day leave to attend the meeting there was a lot
> of excitement about this unusual chance to give users a
> voice. . .further meetings were organized and the group
> formed, participating in training to interview and really getting
> to grips with the nitty-gritty of the project. We were having
> our say and this was being listened to, our ideas being put into
> action. I felt a bit wobbly at times, but ultimately the support of
> the group got me through . . .

On to the interview themselves. . .I found these really enjoyable. Camaraderie developed between the interviewers and it was a dynamic challenge to make sure it came off all right, enabling the person visited to have their say. At times I found it hard to witness the distress of some of the people we interviewed, but hope that through this process we're heading for better-quality services. . .Almost inevitably, I had a relapse before the end of the project. However, I was really touched and heartened by how I was kept informed about how things were going, and as soon as I was well enough I was straight back to interviewing again. (User Focused Monitoring Team 2000)

Mental health service managers had commissioned the project to find out what mental health service users thought of the services. The research commissioners wanted to know how they could make the services more person-centred. To do this, they ensured that each of the tailor-made questionnaires covered the following areas:

- Information
- The care delivery process
- Clinical issues
- Mental health crises
- User involvement
- Advocacy, health record and complaints
- User satisfaction with care.

Two of the project's findings were:

- When asked what was missing from their care, a large number of mental health service users said 'someone to talk to'. Although talking therapies were popular amongst those service users with access to them, what many seemed to want was a 'sympathetic ear' and the chance to talk about ordinary things (Rose 2001, p. 6)
- Isolation was an important issue for mental health service users.

Now take a look at Pause Point 6.4: this asks you to reflect on the value of service-user knowledge.

Pause Point 6.4: The value of service-user knowledge

Identify what it was about the project described above that meant staff changed the services they provided to their clients.

What are your views on what users say about the services you are involved with?

On a scale of 1–10, how would you rate the impact of service-user views on service delivery in your work setting?

If your rating is low (less than 7), make a list of the reasons for this and also list what might be done to improve the impact of service-user views.

To conclude

Across the many different service delivery settings where interprofessional and inter-agency working happens, there is also a need to work with and learn about, from and with the person using services you offer. We called this learning and working together to indicate that learning and working with patients/clients/service users builds on interprofessional learning and working. It is a way of being a student and then being a practitioner that is essential for the effective delivery of services. It requires attending to and valuing what service users know, enabling their knowledge to be heard, then putting what you have learnt in this way to good use in your professional practice.

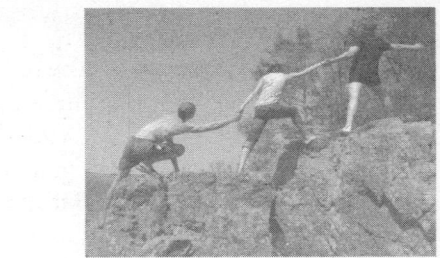

7

Learning About, From and With Carers

Do not wait for leaders; do it alone, person to person.

Mother Teresa

What you will read in this chapter

In Part I of this book, we wrote that being interprofessional was about learning and working with others in certain kinds of ways. We highlighted how being interprofessional means practising in an inclusive way and how learning in anticipation of events rather than just reacting to situations is valuable. In this chapter we demonstrate these aspects of being interprofessional, with a focus on learning about, learning from and learning and working with people who are unpaid carers.

We do this separately from writing about learning and working with service users. This is because we feel that grouping both together can imply that unpaid carers are simply an extension to the person they are caring for. You may have seen this done elsewhere. We are not saying this is wrong. Sometimes it usefully distinguishes all those people who live with an illness or problem (and these are not necessarily the same thing), every day and at home, from those who are responsible for helping with the management of the illness or condition in their work or voluntary role.

In this book, we are focusing on inclusive interprofessional team practices that recognize the distinctiveness, and celebrate the different strengths, of everyone in that team. Unpaid carers are distinct from service users. They bring a different sort of knowledge to the learning team and their contribution to care is unique. In the following pages you will find:

- An exercise to help you learn some of the facts *about* carers in the UK
- Extracts from an article written by a carer *from* her perspective
- A discussion of ways to learn and work *with* carers.

Learning about carers

The diverse settings in which public service delivery teams work mean there is a spectrum of different ways in which children and adults are supported by their family and friends. The example of Timothy in chapter 6 showed just one of those. Much of this support and care is part of our normal responsibility as a parent, partner and friend. Think about the care you provide for others in this way.

You may be a parent and have the responsibility that caring for a child and young person brings. Parental responsibility changes over time. The twenty-four-hour care a baby requires is eventually replaced by a loving but *at-a-distance* relationship with adult children. For most parents, this is how they expected it to be. But, as Timothy's parent discovered, an unexpected illness can change that natural order.

You may care for your parents at the weekend: doing their shopping, putting out what tablets they need to take the following week, or taking a day off work to take them to a hospital appointment. You may have sat with a bereaved friend, supported her as she arranged a funeral, and taken the telephone calls from kindly people she just could not speak to at that time.

You can probably think of other people who you care for and the many other things we all do for each other. Sometimes it is only when this kind of support is missing that we realize how much our family and friends do for us. People in our social networks frequently provide essential support and care; this is something we look at again in chapter 8.

But at certain times in our lives any one of us may need extra care and support from others. Mostly, these episodes are time limited but not always. They may recur and sometimes they can last for months or years. For some people, managing the normal things in their everyday life will always depend on someone else providing physical and /or emotional support.

It is often impossible for people to provide the level of care needed for the time it is needed *and* to do everything else they would normally do in their lives. Something has to go! This can mean a carer changing from full-time to part-time work, or giving up their job completely. Other activities may have to be curtailed: holidays, leisure pursuits and time on their own. In these situations the carer is an integral and important member of the interprofessional team. Carers are often the vital ingredient helping someone to live independently or enabling a person who wants to, to die at home.

Unpaid carers with the roles outlined above are often invisible in

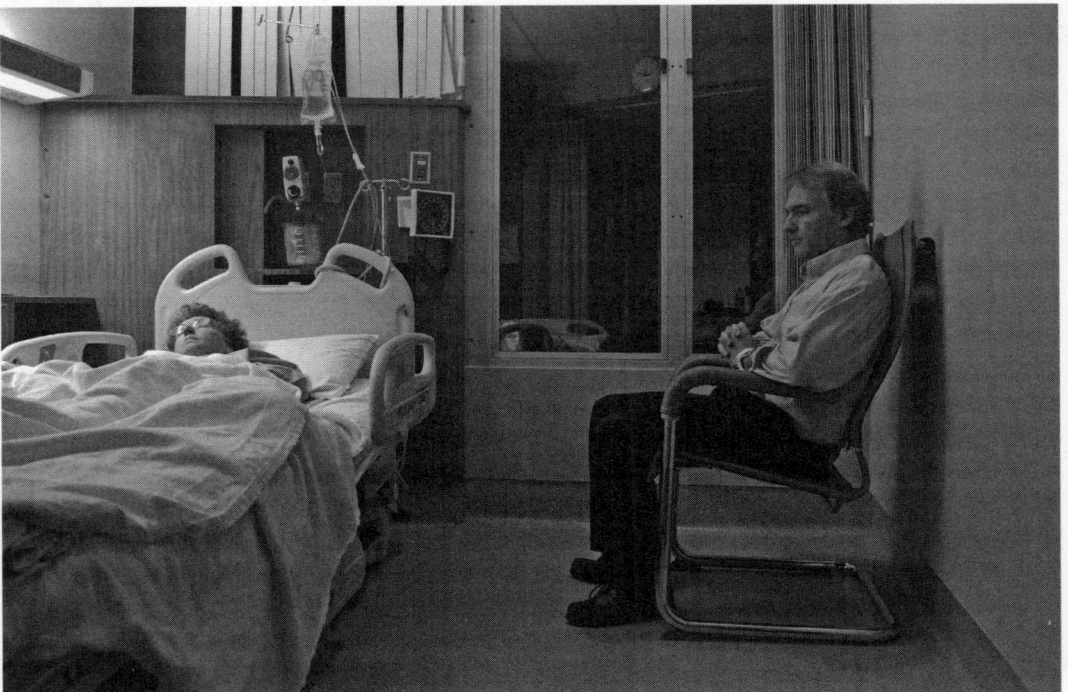

Photo 7.1 Unpaid carers are often invisible; it is important to focus your practice on them as well as the patient or client. Claudio Rossol/ iStock.

the community and to health and social care agencies. Similarly, in schools and workplaces we may not know which of our students or colleagues are also carers. When we do find this out, it can still be difficult to understand what it is like for them to be a carer.

Evidence indicates that sometimes practitioners working in health and social care agencies may be unaware of the work that carers do. It's easy to assume that a service user either somehow manages on their own or that they have someone to help, without realizing how much and what their carer does for them. It's possible for the knowledge and skills that carers develop to be invisible and for their views to be ignored at, for example, case conferences to decide on a client's future care needs.

Finally, the considerable impact of the work of caring on the carer is often unnoticed. Their health and well-being may be affected by the unpaid work they are doing; their social networks may be diminished and their financial, practical and emotional health needs unmet. Sometimes this means that eventually they find it impossible to care for their relative or friend. But they still care about them. This makes relinquishing care to others difficult for the carer and service user.

We think finding out more about carers is an important part

Learner Exercise 7.1: Finding out about carers in the UK

1   Who is a carer? How is this role officially defined?
2   How many people in the UK are carers?
3   How much does unpaid care save the health service?
4   What are the main reasons people need a carer?
5   How many young people are carers?
6   What are good ways to find out who is a young carer?
7   What sort of financial help is available to someone who is a carer?
8   What is a carer's assessment?
9   What rights to an assessment do carers have?
10 Who has the responsibility to carry out a carer's assessment?

Pause Point 7.1: Learning about and from carers in your work

Think of the patients/clients/service users you have recently had contact with; try to identify someone who is unable to always manage their daily life on their own. Take a moment to reflect on the following questions:

Who helps to care for this person?
Have you met the carer?
What would happen if the carer was unable to carry on?
How can you help the carer?
How can the carer help you in your work with this patient/client/service user?

of interprofessional learning, and have designed the questions in Learner Exercise 7.1 to help you with this (the answers to these questions can be found at the end of the chapter). The exercise encourages you to be proactive in your learning about carers. In chapter 5 we distinguished between reactive and proactive learning. This may be a good time to remind yourself about this.

You can do this exercise alone or with a team of interprofessional learners. If necessary, review what we said about team work in chapter 3; perhaps you need to check who is leading the team for this particular exercise. If needed, help with the answers can be found at the following websites: <http://www.carersuk.org/Home>, <http://www.carers.org/> and <http://www.youngcarers.net/>, and there is a good summary about carer's assessments on <www.direct.gov.co.uk>.

When you have finished Learner Exercise 7.1, read Pause Point 7.1. This asks you to relate what you have learnt about carers in general to your practice setting and to a service user you have recently worked with. If you find it hard to identify someone for this, then take the opportunity to work jointly on it with someone from another work setting.

The context of care giving

Caring takes place in a variety of contexts and, as with any human interactions, relationships are not always harmonious. There can be conflicts of interest between the carer's wishes and those of the service user. People who are caring for others also have a variety of other roles – parent, spouse and friend. The emotional and practical interchange between the carers and those they are caring for can be complex; their relationship has its own history and dynamic.

Differences can exist in attitudes to changes in care bought about by new policies. For example, while MIND – the Mental Health Association (<http://www.mind.org.uk>) – campaigned for long-stay mental health-care institutions to be closed down and replaced by community care, SANE (<http://www.sane.org.uk/>), which represents mental health service users and their families, were wary about the impact of the closure of long-stay institutions. As a student or practitioner, being aware that differences like this might occur between service users and their carers is important. You need to support both users and carers as participants in decision-making, and they may have conflicting views on how policies will affect them personally.

Another common conflict between users and carers relates to autonomy, risk-taking and personal safety. Take, for example, an older person who wishes to continue to live in their own home. However, they have become frail, have occasional falls and can be forgetful. Sometimes they forget to turn the gas off and to lock their front door. They do not always answer the telephone so their children, who live some distance away, find it hard to check that they are well. Some carers in this situation will be powerful advocates of their relative's right to live independently in their own homes for as long as possible; others do not want to see their relative exposed to risk and feel that professionals should persuade the older person to accept the *safe* option of residential care.

The Mental Capacity Act (2005) provides guidelines for carers and practitioners about who can take decisions in situations like this. It says that everyone should be treated as able to make their own decisions until it is shown that they can't. It also aims to enable people to make their own decisions for as long as they are capable of and to nominate someone to take decisions for them when they cannot. However, putting this into practice can be complex.

Relationships between carers and practitioners can also be complex. Sometimes practitioners take a negative view of carers, seeing them as putting their own interests before that of their relatives. At other times, practitioners may get drawn into acting on behalf of the carer rather than the service user. In the example above, this may mean they ignore the older person and communicate directly

---

Box 7.1: A conflict in meeting the information needs of a carer

Mrs Y phoned the Scottish Mental Welfare Commission. She was very distressed about the care of her twenty-two-year-old son, who had been admitted to hospital for the second time with what was clearly a psychotic illness. The first admission was voluntary; this one was under a compulsory order. She had a very difficult time trying to look after him after the first admission. He became very negative about her. He was using illicit drugs and alcohol which she thought made him worse. She had been trying to get an appointment to speak to his consultant to get information about his current illness and treatment. However, she had been told that this was impossible for reasons of confidentiality because her son was unwilling to consent to such a discussion.

(Mental Welfare Commission for Scotland 2006, p. 1)

Pause Point 7.2: Sharing information with carers

What does your professional code of conduct say you should do in the circumstances shown in Box 7.1?
In what circumstances can you give information to a carer?
How would you seek to resolve the tension shown in Box 7.1?

---

with the carer (SCIE 2006). So you can see that communicating with both users and carers equitably is an important and complex part of interprofessional practice.

Yet another common tension arises from the need to safeguard the privacy of service users while ensuring the provision of appropriate information to carers. As Box 7.1 shows, this can cause a lot of distress. After reading Mrs Y's story, look at Pause Point 7.2 to relate the challenge of information sharing to your practice setting. Note that we return in detail to this issue in chapter 9.

We have explored some of the tensions that can arise between service users, carers and practitioners. We now briefly touch on the issues of neglect and abuse of service users by carers. Although these happen infrequently, they are particular risks for vulnerable adults and children. The organization Action on Elder Abuse (<www.elderabuse.org.uk>) highlights the neglect and abuse of older people in service, domiciliary and home settings. Children and adults with learning disabilities are also at risk of physical, sexual and emotional abuse in service settings, the community and at home (Brown 1999). There is guidance on multi-agency work to protect vulnerable adults from abuse (Department of Health and the Home Office 2000). Being interprofessional means working collaboratively with carers and being aware of the complexities and tensions associated with this way of working.

Learning from a carer

You should now know a little more about carers and the tensions that may arise for practitioners working with carers, and you will have thought about carers in relation to your own learning and practice. We move on to learning from carers about the work they do, how they feel and how best to work with them.

One way of learning from carers is to listen to what they have to say. In Box 7.2 Monica Clarke, who has been a carer, tells her story about being in this role. Monica teaches us what it's like to be a carer and about her contribution to her husband's care. She also makes the point that the carer is part of the interprofessional team. Does this happen in the place you learn and work in? Take a moment to reflect on the questions in Pause Point 7.3. You might also like to consider what Monica says about the evidence base for caring. She points out this is not found in the way that evidence is usually found in the social

---

Box 7.2: Monica Clarke, an ex-carer writes . . .

Emphasis needs to be taken away from the carer as a receiver of services, and placed on the capabilities, skills and knowledge which they contribute to the team as equals.

The needs of the carer are often seen as relating to the well-being of the cared for: almost as if they are connected by an extended umbilical cord, without a separate identity of their own. Looking at the carer as part of the workforce can potentially cut this cord and allow the carer to develop as an individual.

I nursed my husband, who was being fed through a tummy tube (gastrostomy) for many years. Although he was paralysed on one side, he did not allow us to clean his tummy around the tube: that was his private place and only he was allowed to touch the saline swab and clean around the tube. All of us caring for him – the home support workers included – respected this. However, when the district nurse came, she put on her sterile gloves, jacked up his pyjamas, got her saline swab out and got to work – without asking his permission, without waiting to see how it is usually done at home. Is it any wonder that my husband slapped her on the wrist and growled at her through his aphasic anger?

As a carer, and after many years being an observer of how health professionals work, I know that I can reflect back to them the good practice of some of their colleagues – if only I could be allowed an equal place around the professional table, to pass on to them the knowledge I have gained.

We can all bring our different expertise to the table to get a better overall result. They would bring to me the care prescribed by their professional regulators. I would bring to them the actual care delivered at home, and together, with the cared for, we could map out an agreed path of care which incorporates all our desired outcomes.

The evidence base of caring lies outside that which usually governs health and social sciences, which rely on the philosophy of rational, systematic, scientific structure. Caring, though, is difficult to define and evaluate with this way of thinking as it is based on phenomenology, that is, on the meaning of the relationships, on art: on creativity and innovation, on working around and within undefined circumstances.

Escalation of the skills of the family carer is vital to the success of care in the community. It is vital that the presence of the carer be embraced, in practice, within the *professional of interprofessional*. Then the carer would no longer be seen as an extension of the cared for, who acts only as a reactor to the requirements of other disciplines. Then we would be respected in our own right, and we will be given our rightful place within the shared learning experience.

This is adapted from 'The Family Carer as Part of the Interprofessional Team',
originally published in the *CAIPE Bulletin Issue* (29 January 2008):
it is reproduced here with permission from the author and CAIPE

Pause Point 7.3: The carers in your interprofessional team

Think again of the carer you identified in Pause Point 7.1

What are the best ways of enabling this carer to be part of the interprofessional care team?
What barriers might there be to this?
What can you and your colleagues do to overcome these barriers?
How best can the interprofessional team learn from the carer?

and health sciences. It is more likely to be found by exploring the phenomenon of being a carer and through creative ways of collecting data. Monica's story is itself an example of this, and we turn to another role for the arts in our section on learning with carers that ends this chapter.

Learning with carers

Involving carers in education and training and staff development activities is a powerful way for the interprofessional team to learn from their insights. Practitioners need to understand more of what a carer knows about the person they care for and what they do for that person. Reading carers' stories and listening to them at team meetings is likely to help you to do this. But sometimes this is not quite enough.

In chapter 1 we wrote how being interprofessional involves knowing what to do, how to do it and having the right attitudes about this way of practising. Our attitudes are related to our emotions, to what it feels like to act in a certain way or to be in a certain role. You will recall that we wrote about emotional intelligence and the part it can play in effective team-working in chapter 3. We think it is important to understand how it feels to be a carer and to appreciate the emotions carers experience as they undertake their role.

So, ideally, learning with carers should enable practitioners to have some insight into carers' feelings. We have an example of this in Box 7.3, with the work of a UK council. The staff from the council worked with carers to meet social services staff development needs. Together, they devised and delivered an interprofessional learning initiative. This not only bought together practitioners and carers; it called on the professional expertise of arts practitioners for a way of facilitating learning that included learning about emotions. Lots of interprofessional collaboration in one initiative!

Note that this happened because staff identified their learning

---

Box 7.3: Staff development work with carers in Doncaster, UK

Doncaster Council's Community and Carers Development Team carried out a review of adult social care practice in relation to carers' assessments in June 2006, prompted by the need to improve the local authority's performance. During the review, staff specifically asked for training about carers; therefore one of the key recommendations of the report was the provision of training sessions about carers' legislation, carers' rights and carers' issues for all adult social care staff.

The Community and Carers Development Team was keen to find a creative way of delivering training to social care practitioners that would raise awareness of informal carers and their needs. Doncaster Arts (darts) was approached, and they agreed to train the Community and Carers Development Team in constructing a piece of forum theatre that showed the different pressures faced by informal carers.

In forum theatre, the audience ('spect-actors') watch a short play that shows a character being oppressed. The play is then repeated exactly as it was done the first time, with the actors trying to bring the play to the same end as before. Members of the audience try to change the ending to break the oppression and show that new solutions are possible. When the play is running for a second time, the spect-actors can shout 'stop' and then either give suggestions or take over the actor's role to try and change the ending themselves. The game is spect-actors – trying to find a new solution – against the actors, who are trying to hold them back, to force them to accept the world as it is. The spect-actors, by acting out their ideas, train for 'real-life' action and are spurred into finding new solutions and inventing new ways of confronting oppression.

In August 2007 darts worked with the team over six days, showing them how to construct a piece of forum theatre using the issues identified by carers, and then teaching them how to facilitate it. The piece of theatre was to be performed by the team at training sessions for social care practitioners.

The final play told the story of Carol, who was struggling to care for her mum, Doreen, and still find time for herself and the rest of her family; it illustrated the need for the social worker involved to take into account Carol's needs and not just Doreen's. The Community and Carers Development Team hoped that the play would 'give the audience a different perspective of a situation they see on a daily basis'.

The story was developed from a series of meetings that the Community and Carers Development Team had with carers in Doncaster. Staff from the team talked individually to the carers about their caring role, then asked them to describe the ways in which this had impacted on them as individuals and in particular how they felt about this. It was important to pick up on the feelings, as these feelings would be acted out to the audience.

The forum theatre was one element of a training programme that was delivered over two days. To develop the programme, staff talked to a separate group of carers to find out what they wanted social care practitioners to know about carers. One of the things carers wanted the practitioners to know was how it really feels to be a carer, hence the forum theatre.

The social care practitioners who took part in the forum theatre described the play as 'powerful and thought-provoking', said that 'it highlighted both the client and carer's issues' and 'added real emotion to the subject.' They described the practical element of the forum as 'interactive and innovative', and 'a very interesting and unusual approach', and thought forum theatre was an 'excellent learning tool'.

The staff invited a carer along to watch the forum theatre and give a reality check from the carer's perspective. The carer's response was that it was true to real life.

This interactive approach to looking at the role of the carer seemed to capture audiences' imagination and led to some very interesting debates about how social care services could find new solutions to caring for the carer.

The Community and Carers Development Team are keen to continue with this creative method in future training to raise awareness of carers' issues, and to keep carers involved in the process.

(Adapted from a review of adult social care practice in relation to carers' assessments by Doncaster Council's Community and Carers Development Team in June 2006)

needs about carers: this is an important initial step in reactive learning. The staff also commented on the way the theatre piece highlighted *emotional* issues. The feedback from practitioners who experienced the forum theatre in Box 7.3 indicated how important this was in enabling a full understanding of the carer in the interprofessional team.

Some key points about learning and working with carers are:

- The carer is an equal in the interprofessional team
- Their knowledge has an equal part to play in decision-making about how care is delivered
- Carers and the person they care for have separate identities.

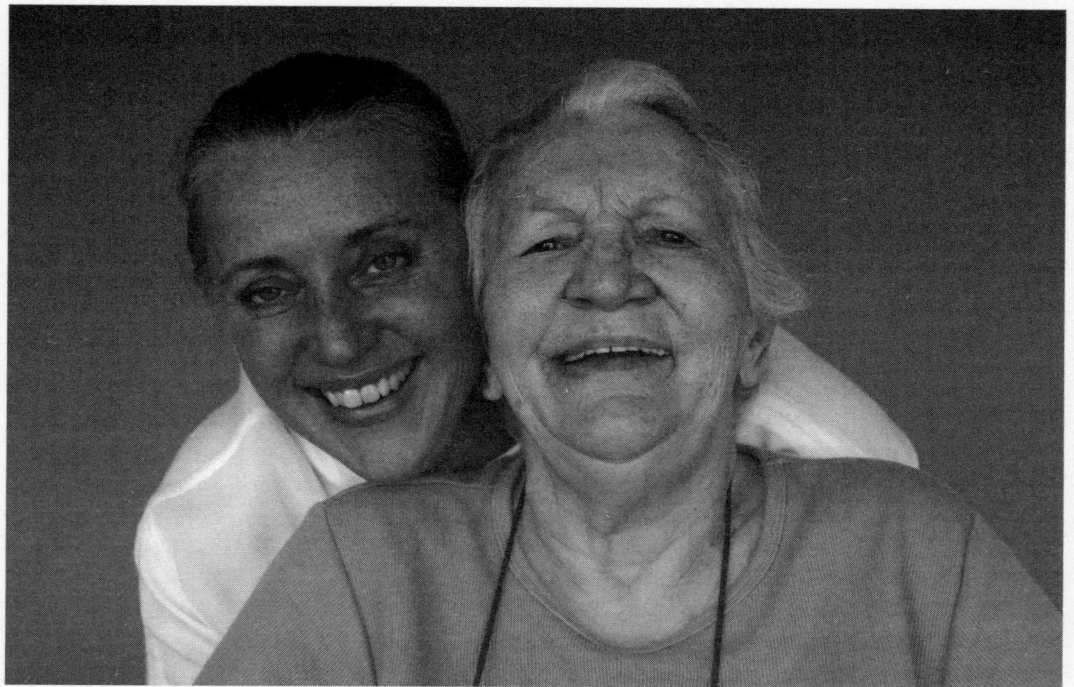

Photo 7.2 Carers and the person they care for have separate identities. Cliff Parnell/iStock.

You may be able to add more from your experiences with carers of people in your practice area, or perhaps from your work with young carers.

To conclude

Effective services depend on everyone's contribution and upon everyone learning about each other, from each other, and learning and working with each other. This chapter has emphasized the important part that carers have in collaborative working and in enabling new understandings about practice and service delivery.

The value in learning about, from and with carers extends in many cases from informal and often unrecognized learning opportunities, to actively involving them in learning opportunities for professional practitioners in similar ways to those presented in this chapter.

Answers to the questions in Learner Exercise 7.1

1   Carers provide care for others on an *unpaid* basis; so this excludes paid care workers, home helps and people employed by

someone with a disability. A carer's allowance is a taxable benefit to help people who look after someone who is disabled. You do not have to be related to, or live with, the person that you care for. (For more information, see: <http://www.direct.gov.uk/en/CaringForSomeone/MoneyMatters/DG_10012522>.)

2   In 2001, Carers UK said that:

In any one year, 301,000 adults in the UK become carers.

Over a lifetime, seven out of ten women will be carers, and nearly six out of ten men.

Women have a fifty-fifty chance of having substantial caring responsibilities by the time they are fifty-nine. Men have the same chance aged seventy-four.

We currently have a 6.6 per cent chance in any one year of becoming a carer.

1.7 million carers provide over twenty hours of care per week.

3   In 2008, the average person caring for a sick or frail relative is now estimated to save the UK health service more than £15,260 per person a year. This is based on the cost of alternative care at £14.50 an hour.

4   Because due to age, physical or mental illness, addiction or disability they cannot mange their lives without some help.

5   Of all those aged eighteen to twenty-four, 4 per cent will have regularly cared for an ill or disabled relative during their own childhood.

6   If you work with adults, some probably have a care need because of their disability, illness or substance mis-use problem. Think about who else looks after your client. Tens of thousands say their child is also their carer. To find out about children who are carers, you need only to ask every adult client or patient:

- Who helps care for you at home?
- Do you have children?
- What effect does your health problem have on them?
- How much do they do to help out?
- Do you need more support as a parent?
- Do your children need more support?

7   A carer's allowance is the main state benefit, but more may be available to people on low incomes.

8   A carer's assessment would discuss the help that a carer needed with caring, plus the help they needed to maintain their own health and to balance caring with their own life, work and family commitments. The assessment is used to decide what practical, financial and other help to provide. Many carers do not know they have a right to this assessment – has the carer you know of had an assessment? A good introduction to a carer's assessment is available from Carers UK on: <http://www.carersuk.org/Information/Helpwithcaring/Carersassessmentguide>.

9   Carers have a legal right to an assessment: see the Carers (Equal Opportunities) Act 2004 available at: <http://www.opsi.gov.uk/acts/acts2004>.
10 The local authority; by a social worker or a member of social services.

The authors are grateful to Monica Clarke for giving permission to publish her article and to Liz George for her help in compiling the section about the forum theatre.

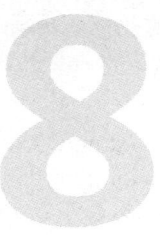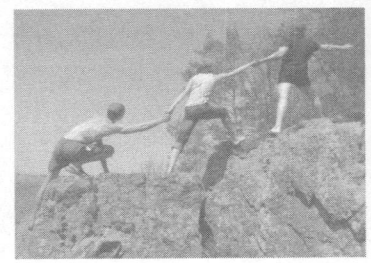

The Statutory, Community, Voluntary and Private Sectors: Learning About, From and With Each Other

Give to every human being every right that you claim for yourself.
Robert Ingersoll

What you will read in this chapter

This chapter focuses on interprofessional relationships between statutory, voluntary, community and private-sector staff, and on why these are important to your practice. You will see that many of the skills you use in other interprofessional work apply in this wider and increasingly important context. The practice-related examples we use show that relationships across these different sectors can work well. On the other hand, the voluntary and community sector perspectives can be challenging to those working in the statutory sector. With the increasing provision of social and health-care services by private companies, it becomes more and more likely that you may collaborate with colleagues from organizations that are run with a commercial intent.

All these sectors provide important support to service users. With that in mind this chapter considers:

- The contributions that the statutory, voluntary, community and private sectors make to interprofessional working
- Strategies for building relationships across the sectors
- The importance of interprofessional networks in the context of social inclusion.

The contribution of diverse sectors to effective services

There is increasing recognition that networking across diverse sectors is important to the provision of effective services. No one practitioner, agency or sector on its own can see the whole picture, particularly in areas of complex practice. We start with an inspiring example of voluntary, community and statutory sector working. Box 8.1 shows the vital role and the great value to staff and service users

---

Box 8.1: The role and value of a voluntary sector organization

I cannot imagine delivering services without the help of the Cleft Lip and Palate Association (CLAPA). I am on their executive board and they have representatives on our management boards. Each of the eight cleft palate centres in the UK has a cleft lip and palate association loosely attached to it.

CLAPA sent a questionnaire to parents about their experience of using health services. It asked them what the gaps were. They found that until parents managed to get to specialist services they were not getting much information from nurses and midwives about feeding and breathing for babies with difficulties. Parents had to struggle to get to a cleft centre, and that was taking six to eight months at a crucial time in a child's life. This led to the reorganization of services and the development of the nurse specialist role. Now they get a contact with a specialist centre within forty-eight hours of a diagnosis. CLAPA supply the specialist feeding equipment once the nurse specialist has made the initial assessment and we recommend to parents that they contact CLAPA for parent mentor support.

When we see parents we give them an information pack with CLAPA's leaflets in – they produce good parent-centred information and their information is accurate! There is a lot of misleading information out there on the Internet – so we always refer them to CLAPA's website.

For these people, what voluntary services offer is different from statutory services. There can be a 'we know' feeling in statutory services, but it is important to recognize that sometimes the only people who know what something feels like are the people who have been through it. A lot of things are best coming from people who have experienced what it was like for them – for example, your child being diagnosed with a cleft palate in pregnancy, or if your baby has feeding and breathing problems from a Pierre Robin sequence airways obstruction and they need a breathing tube. This places an enormous burden of care on the families. Seeing a happy three-year-old who has been through health difficulties and come out the other side can give more hope and optimism to parents than any amount of reassurance from practitioners.

CLAPA are currently developing their website – <www.clapa.com> – to include chatrooms for children and an interactive one to bring teenagers together.

It's a wonderful organization and we couldn't do without it.

of the Cleft Lip and Palate Association (CLAPA) (<http://www.clapa.com>) in the words of Alison, a cleft palate nurse specialist team leader. In Pause Point 8.1 there are some questions related to Alison's commentary – take a few moments to reflect on these, on your own or with other students.

Pause Point 8.1: Working with people with experience

- Who benefits from the collaboration between voluntary sector and statutory sectors?
- What advantages does Alison see in working with CLAPA?

The theme of sharing experiences with someone who has 'been there' is one which recurs in many accounts of community and voluntary sector organizations.

- How might people who use the service in your area of practice meet with those who have had similar experiences?
- What organizations exist to help these service users?

We learnt from Alison (Box 8.1) how nursing staff employed in an organization in the statutory sector (the health service) work collaboratively with staff from a voluntary organization. As the title of this chapter indicates, the community sector and private companies also provide services to people with social and health-care needs. All these sectors have essential and different characteristics and roles that are better understood by knowing a little more about them. Because voluntary and community sector organizations are diverse, we also comment briefly on some different types of organizations.

The statutory sector

In the UK, the powers and responsibilities of the statutory agencies are defined by statute and enshrined in law. Funding is ongoing, although not necessarily always maintained at the same level from year to year. Budgets are ultimately set by central government. The career paths of staff working in statutory sector organizations tend to be more defined than those in other sectors. These organizations are usually hierarchical with clear management structures and lines of accountability. Health authorities, education authorities, local authorities and the police are all statutory organizations.

The voluntary and community sectors

This sector includes a wide range of organizations, from large and very well-known national charities to small local groups. Internationally, they are often collectively referred to as non-

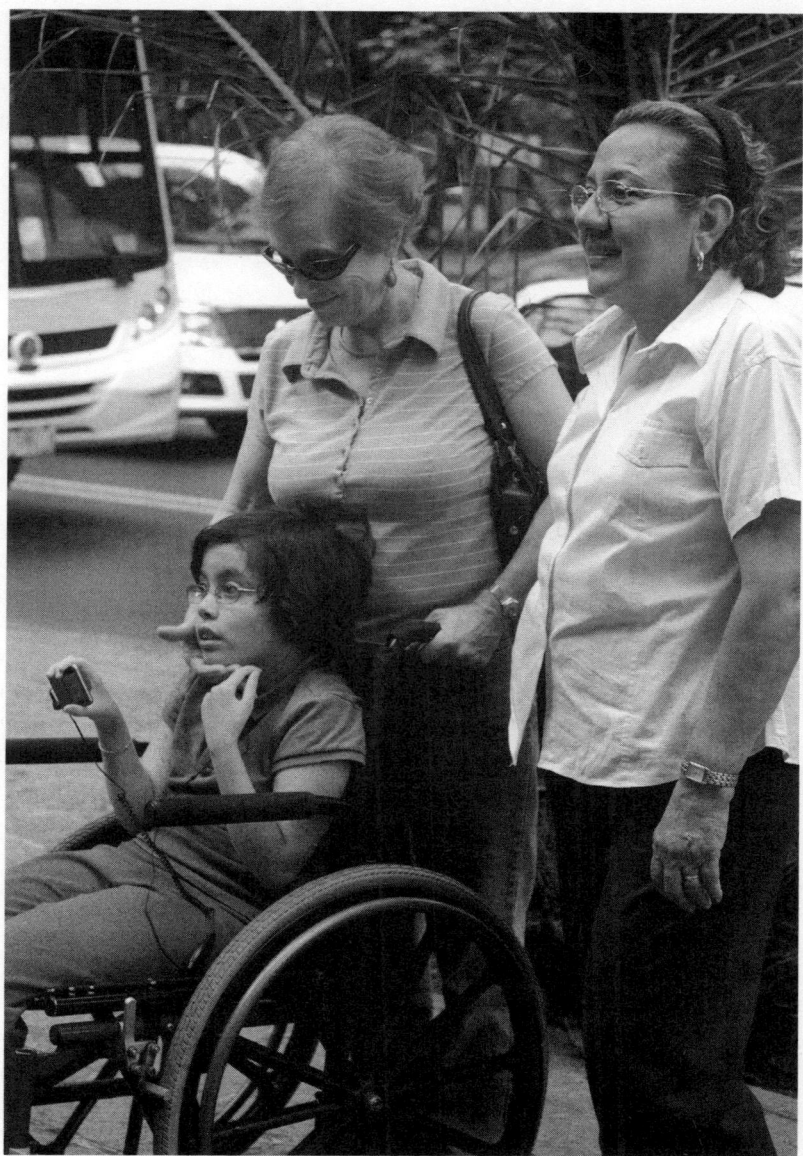

Photo 8.1 The voluntary sector includes large organizations such as Age Concern, as well as smaller, locally run social groups, to offer support to people in the community. Andres balcazar/iStock.

governmental organizations or NGOs. Sometimes, in the UK, they are known as the third sector. Included in this category are large organizations such as Shelter, Age Concern and Mind (National Association for Mental Health). These have million-pound budgets and a head office, and some have local offices all around the country. Others, for example, an Asian women's refuge and some religious organizations, are likely to be smaller and dependent upon one or two workers. Some smaller organizations run purely on voluntary effort, such as a local mothers' and toddlers' group or a resident's association. While some organizations, like CLAPA, see themselves as complementing the statutory sector, others are more challenging and might aim to provide alternative services: some do both.

In general, all these organizations (large and small) have been created freely in response to a perceived need. That need may have been local, national, client group or issue related. They are normally grant aided or funded through subscriptions and donations. Some are run by volunteers; others employ staff. Management varies from organization to organization. A local group will often have a steering group made up of local people, while the larger organizations might have a management structure and trustees. In the UK, many of these organizations will be registered as charities with the Charities Commission, and thus able to take advantage of certain tax exemptions permitted to charities.

Learner Exercise 8.1 is designed to help you get to know two voluntary organizations better and to identify more about their roles as service providers. We think our choices (Age Concern and MIND)

Learner Exercise 8.1: Looking more closely at voluntary organizations

Age Concern for older people and MIND (National Association for Mental Health) are two large well-known UK voluntary organizations.

Note your answers here

Have a look at their websites:

- Age Concern <www.ageconcern.org.uk>
- MIND <www.mind.org.uk>

What kind of help do they offer?
What do they see as their role?
Are there differences between the roles of CLAPA, Age Concern and MIND?

Age Concern and MIND both highlight the issues of stigma and discrimination in relation to their service users.

What else are they concerned about?
What else do Age Concern and MIND have in common?
What do they not offer?
What ways might you use these organizations in your work?

are relevant to almost every area of practice. If this is not the case, then select two other large and similar voluntary organizations that feel more relevant to your practice. This is another learner exercise that you might choose to do firstly by yourself and then with other students in the interprofessional team. We suggested earlier that if you are on a practice placement, one way of doing this is to find one or more students from other professions who are allocated to the same place, and to do the exercise with them. Look at any differences between the answers when you did the exercise by yourself and when you did it with others.

Self-help groups

Some self-help groups fit easily into the category of voluntary and community organizations described above: others are harder to categorize. We've chosen two examples. The first shows how a small self-help organization – SANDS – can effect a big change in practice (Box 8.2); the second shows how one self-help organization, Alcoholics Anonymous (AA), has become a role model for other twelve-step programmes (Box 8.3). If you go to the AA website you can find some of the answers to the questions we ask you to consider in Pause Point 8.3

(<http://www.alcoholics-anonymous.org.uk/geninfo/05step. htm>; accessed August 2008).

Box 8.2: An overview of the impact of SANDS

The Stillbirth and Neonatal Death Society (SANDS) is a UK national charity, established in 1981 by bereaved parents to:

Support anyone affected by the death of a baby.
Work in partnership with health practitioners to **improve the quality of care** and services offered to bereaved families.
Promote research and **changes in practice** that could help to reduce the loss of babies' lives.

Prior to 1981, when a baby died in hospital at or after birth their body was usually taken away. The baby's parents would often not know what had happened to it. In some extreme cases body parts were used without consent. Parents did not get the opportunity to name, or see or bury their baby. This resulted in distressed parents at the time or afterwards. Many practitioners thought that what they were doing was in the best interests of parents. After a campaign by bereaved parents this practice changed. Current good practice guidelines were drawn up jointly by parents and health practitioners, and parents can choose whether to name and bury their baby.

(More information can be found at <http://www.uk-sands.org>)

Take a moment to read Pause Points 8.2 and 8.3, as they follow on from Boxes 8.2 and 8.3: each asks for some reflection on collaboration between self-help groups and statutory sector practitioners.

Box 8.3: Alcoholics Anonymous and twelve-step programmes: a brief outline

One of the largest growths of self-help movements has been through the twelve-step programme used first by Alcoholics Anonymous (AA). AA was established in the 1930s in the United States of America. One of its founders was Bill Wilson, a Wall Street banker whose career was ruined by drunkenness. Members' primary purpose is to stay sober and help other alcoholics to achieve sobriety.

There are now twelve-step programmes which deal with different kinds of addiction. These include drug abuse, gambling and eating difficulties. They are often an important source of support and might form part of a service user's network. For more information, see <http://www.12step.org>.

Pause Point 8.2: Reflecting on the work of SANDS

Why do you think many practitioners resisted the change?
Can you think of any changes that are being campaigned for today?
What is it like to hear criticism of the way that you work?

Pause Point 8.3: Reflecting on the role of Alcoholics Anonymous

Why do you think this group and others based on a similar model are so popular?
What is distinctive about their philosophy?
What do they offer people that is not offered by the statutory services?

Activist organizations

These are organizations set up by people to campaign for change. They are usually concerned with changing an aspect of policy or legislation, or highlighting a particular issue. There is often an overlap of activist work with that of voluntary and community sector organizations. Often, though, activists use different tactics and have a point of view that may challenge mainstream opinions.

Many large and well-established non-statutory organizations were started by a few activists. Shelter, for example, was set up in the 1960s by some activists who were concerned about homelessness. Have a look at their website: <www.england.shelter.org.uk>. Some activist

Box 8.4: Self-help as a way of being heard

The Scottish Dementia Working Group was set up by some people with dementia in Scotland, who were concerned that their voices were not being heard in decision-making and that people experiencing dementia were not seen as able to speak for themselves. They felt that all people with dementia were being lumped together. Anyone who has dementia can become a member and members can bring a carer to the meeting with them if they want. The first time one of them went to a conference about dementia they had to pose as a photographer to get in! Now they sit on decision-making boards.

(<http://www.alzscot.org/pages/sdwg/aboutus.htm>; August 2008)

organizations like Scottish Dementia (Box 8.4) only allow people who have experienced something themselves to join. The kinds of challenges that activist groups raise can be uncomfortable to begin with, but they can have a powerful role influencing service provision, policy and eventually legislation.

The private sector

In the United Kingdom, the provision of social and health-care services by privately run companies has a history and an important current and future role. It is not the place of this book to review history; what we want to do is signal aspects of current and future public service provision that will impact on the working practice of students and staff.

There is a developing and diverse role for commercial organizations that provide health and social care. This change in the balance of services provided by statutory and private sector services means that as a qualified practitioner you may work for a private company, and if you work in the statutory sector you may need to work collaboratively with colleagues from the private sector.

The National Health Service (NHS) provides health-care services free at the point of delivery; social care services are most generally provided according to the means that people have to pay. As with all generalities there are exceptions. For example, private eye care is paid for at the point of delivery by most people of working age; private health care is available for people with the means to pay for it, and older people able to pay may choose to live in privately run sheltered accommodation that (amongst other services) provides warden assistance when emergencies arise. In chapter 4 we wrote about how Lindy moved into a private nursing home after her stroke when she was discharged from the NHS hospital. In England, depending on her financial circumstances, Lindy would have had to pay the fees for her nursing home care: fee-paying rules for such care vary in other parts of the UK.

> **Box 8.5: Examples of social and health services provision by the private sector**
>
> NHS services such as cleaning and catering are contracted out to private companies.
> Adoption services are provided by private state-licensed agencies.
> Occupational health services for statutory sector staff are provided by commercial organizations.
> Private companies offer psychotherapy and counselling services; some of this may be funded by statutory services.
> Privately run pathology services advertise themselves as available to NHS patients.
> Mobility and daily living aids are mostly sold by private companies, often with money supplied from the public purse.
> You may be given a prescription to exercise at your local (privately run) gym by your NHS doctor.
> Resuscitation training courses are mostly provided by private companies.

This paints a simple picture of the balance of statutory and private sector provision. Currently, in reality, it is far more complex. Privately run companies provide many different services across the width of services funded from central and local government (Box 8.5).

There are also less obvious ways in which private companies offer services to enhance well-being and enable people to lead the life they want whatever their circumstances. Examples here include shop-mobility, cloth nappy services and stop-smoking advice, available in local pharmacies – you can probably add items of relevance to your practice to this list and the one in Box 8.5.

Finally, and again briefly, current reforms of UK health care include the capacity for key services to be run by private companies. In its 2002 publication, *Growing Capacity: A New Role for External Healthcare Providers in England*, the government announced 'a new sector in health care provision in England, additional to existing publicly-owned NHS health care provision' (Department of Health 2002). This new style of provision includes treatment and diagnostic units run by independent operators; units that you may refer your clients and patients to and where you may have referrals from. You may also work with staff who work in and people who use treatment centres. Some of these are run by the NHS; some by the independent sector, that is, jointly between the NHS and a private health-care provider. These are just two examples of change; there are likely to be many more across public services in the future.

Collaborative working across different sectors

In the opening sections of this chapter we introduced many different organizations from the voluntary and community sectors, and looked at the role of private companies in the provision of health and social care. Staff working in the statutory sector work and learn with colleagues from these types of organizations and groups as part of their everyday practice. Chapter 5 focused on the centrality of learning and working collaboratively with colleagues within a sector, and chapters 6 and 7 focused on users of services and carers. Put together like this, our list of those who might be learning and working with each other may appear like a patchwork – a patchwork with the potential to fall apart at the seams. This does sometimes happen, as our reference in chapter 4 to the death of Victoria Climbié shows. But it is not always the case. It is possible for organizations and people to work together, to learn about, from and with each other as they work. Our opening example in this chapter demonstrated this. We turn now to some other examples to highlight a few of the issues and challenges in being interprofessional in this patchwork world of delivering services.

Domestic violence: whose business?

Women's Aid organizations were set up in the 1970s by women to highlight domestic violence as a problem, and to campaign for refuges for women and children. At that time domestic violence was often not treated seriously. For example, rape within marriage was not illegal. Refuge and the National Women's Aid Federation now provide services such as a domestic violence helpline, and campaign about domestic violence. They ask everyone to act until women and children are safe – to admit domestic abuse is a problem, call it by its name and talk to someone about it. They have influenced the way domestic violence is treated by the police and health and social care services, and, collaboratively with other organizations, have influenced legislation. Their websites give a history and you can read people's stories on them: <www.womensaid.org.uk> and <www.refuge.org.uk>.

Although not all domestic violence is male to female, one in four women will experience domestic violence at some point in their lives, and one third of domestic violence starts or intensifies when women are pregnant. Many women are victims for many years before they seek help.

> Violence undermines women's health and well-being, directly and indirectly, causing chronic morbidity, increased depression, lower birth weight, and mortality. Among children, witnessing abuse can lead to increased delinquency and gang violence. Overall, violence contributes to reduced quality of life of families and communities and decreased participation by women in the democratic process.'(Duvvery et al. 2004, p. 4)

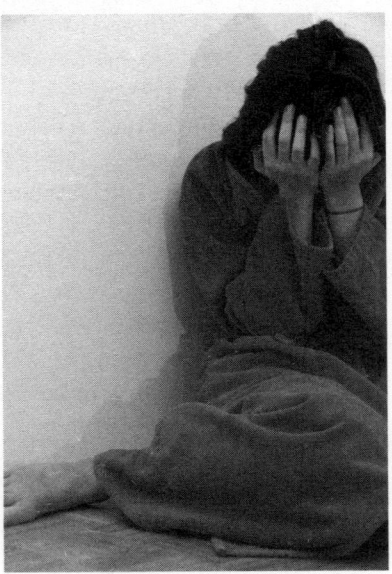

Photo 8.2 Domestic violence is a very complex situation and offers many challenges to effective service provision. Andrija Kovač/iStock.

Domestic violence has an impact on many aspects of the lives of the victims and their families (see Box 8.6 and the quote from Duvvery et al., above).

Domestic violence is an issue for agencies from all the sectors we focus on in this chapter. It involves the police, the law, medical services, refuges, counselling, social work, education, education services, the voluntary sector, families and communities (and this is an abbreviated list). Local areas are increasingly setting up multi-agency domestic violence forums under the auspices of the Crime and Disorder Act (1998) to exchange information between agencies such as the police, social services, health, education and the voluntary sector, and to ensure that maximum protection is given to victims. Routine enquiry about domestic violence is now a part of midwifery practice and all human services workers are asked to be alert to it. This means that, whatever your practice area, identifying who might be a victim of domestic violence is part of your role. Your experience of interprofessional education is planned so that, for example, you know which of your colleagues you can discuss any concerns you have about a patient or client who you think is at risk of domestic violence.

The role and importance of information about services provided by all sectors

With so many services providers in different sectors it can be difficult for people to find out where and who to go to for support. Although we live in the 'information age', sometimes it is hard to get good and reliable targeted information when you want it. This is particularly true if you are in a vulnerable position or a health/emotional crisis. Service users often identify information as being particularly important; they highlight the need for:

- More information about services
- More information about conditions/their situation and its implications for the future
- More information about choices that might be available to help them
- More information about the kinds of support available to them
- More information about their rights, including welfare rights.

(Coulter et al. 1999)

To be useful, information has to be timely, appropriate and accessible. As a practitioner, you are in a position to build up knowledge over time about the kinds of organizations that might complement the work you are doing, and to help service users access information about them. Using a range of information sources, including those put together by people who have experienced vulnerability themselves, can be helpful. Look at Pause Point 8.4 and consider how this might enhance your practice.

Pause Point 8.4: Knowledge about the patient's experience

Have a look at DIPEx.org – this is a site for patient experiences.

Can you think of any ways in which this might complement the work you are doing? Are there any experiences on this website that are familiar to you?

Learner Exercise 8.2 and the story of Ngosi and her family in Case Study 8.1 focus on how to recognize and meet service users' information needs. If you are learning and working with an interprofessional team, try doing the exercise together and comparing

Learner Exercise 8.2: Meeting a service user's information needs

1 Read about Ngosi and her family (Case Study 8.1).

   What are Ngosi's needs and her strengths?
   Where would you suggest she looks for help?
   What kinds of services and organizations might be useful to her? What about the
      communication issues?
   Are there any networks that you might want to find out about?

2 Now think about your practice setting.

   What kind of information is displayed in your waiting room?
   Is it displayed in different formats for people with disabilities/who speak a range
      of languages?
   Can you think of other kinds of information that might be useful to the people
      who wait in this room?

   Finally, find out if your practice setting has a directory of services that are
available locally for the client group you work with.

Case Study 8.1: Ngosi and her family

Ngosi has four children. The youngest is now profoundly deaf after having
meningitis when she was three years old. Ngosi's husband is finding their
daughter's sudden disability difficult to deal with, and Ngosi is trying to find
out as much as possible to help with this and to help her daughter. Her church
group want to help but they don't know what to do. Ngosi wants information
about how to care for her daughter, where she can get support from and about
resources to help her and the rest of the family communicate with her child. She
has had to cut down her work hours since this has happened and feels that a
break for her and the rest of her family is important. All the family, parents and
other children, are feeling the strain.

---

results. This should give you an insight into the different strengths
your colleagues bring to collaborative working.

Finding local information: local compacts and other sources

Local compacts are working agreements between voluntary and
statutory organizations in specific areas, which set out how the
sectors should work with each other. For example, the London
Borough of Kensington and Chelsea has a compact with black
and ethnic minority organizations in the borough. Have a look
at their website: <http://www.westminster-pct.nhs.uk/diversity/
bmehealthforum.htm>. Local compacts can be a good starting

point to finding out what voluntary and community sector organizations are in your area and how they might contribute to your work. Try to answer these questions:

- Is there a compact in your area?
- Who is in it?
- What kind of organizations are in the compact?
- What work does the compact do?

Other good sources of information about local voluntary and community sectors are: the organization called Community Service Volunteers (for more information, see <http://www.csv.org.uk>); Local Authority Children's and Adult Plans; and Local Public Health Reports. It is possible that the client group you work with also has a national self-help group and organization. In chapter 4 we highlighted how agencies and organizations influence working together in teams. The following section looks at how this type of partnership work across different sectors becomes reality.

Building effective partnerships: the Supporting People initiatives

Supporting People is a government programme in England which aims to provide housing-related support to help vulnerable people stay in their own homes, and to increase their independence and capacity for self-care. Supporting People is a working partnership of local government, service users and support agencies. It is also concerned with tackling social exclusion for groups of people who are often marginalized from society. Early work in the Supporting People programme that brought housing, health and social care agencies together indicated that:

- Integrating services to support vulnerable people works best when the service is determined by the needs of the people who use the service rather than by what services already exist
- Voluntary organizations are less constrained by organizational priorities and professional agendas
- Voluntary agencies were more able to respond flexibly to the needs of the individual.

The discussions about some of the challenges to partnership working for organizations and agencies show that these are similar to the ones the individual practitioners face working interprofessionally. They include:

- Different ways of working
- Different priorities
- Issues about confidentiality
- Personal and professional accountability.

Many of the case studies in this chapter and others highlight these challenges. We suggest you read the case studies with this in mind and think about ways in which they might be overcome. A lot can be achieved by building effective partnerships and some ways this is done are discussed in the following sections.

Building effective partnerships: networking

We do not exist in isolation and networks are crucial to all of our lives – whether they are friendship networks, social networks, support networks, networks of interest or local networks. Networking recognizes that people live in a social context and can be an important way of building social capital. Social capital is the sum of all the social networks and connections in a given neighbourhood that an individual can draw on (Giddens 2006).

As a practitioner, it's important for you to understand the social networks of people you are working with and to support them through provision of good information. This will help them to understand what is available to them from public services and can signpost the support available to strengthen their coping strategies. In turn, this enhances their social capital at what might be a vulnerable point in their lives.

Evidence indicates that the more socially excluded people are, the less strong their networks are likely to be. For example, isolation is a major issue faced by many people who are mentally distressed, as well as by people who experience higher rates of violence and harassment against them than rates for people in the general population (Ward 1993). Isolation is a key issue for many older people. Poverty also makes it difficult for people on low incomes to take advantage of the things that many of us take for granted. All of this has a negative impact on their health. See Box 8.7 for more comments on this. Helping people to build social capital can reverse this and lead to increased well-being.

It is the poorest people who come into most contact with the controlling aspects of the state. For example, they are more likely to depend on benefits, and much more likely to have their children taken into care. For these people in particular, networking is crucial. Disenfranchised people are also often those most unlikely to use mainstream services and to be stigmatized by staff providing these services, for example:

- Black young men are disproportionately held in prisons and in secure psychiatric settings, and are more likely to be diagnosed with schizophrenia than their white counterparts
- Refugees and asylum seekers are more likely to be wary of statutory services
- Working-class patients in the UK ask their general practitioner fewer questions and spend less time with the doctor than middle-

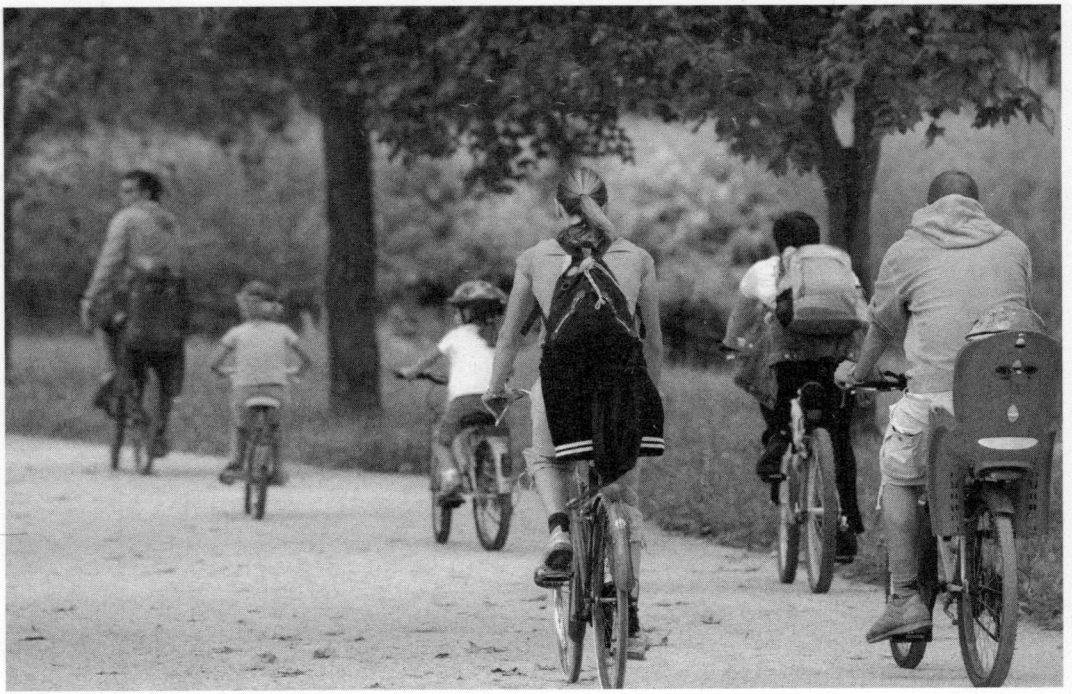

Photo 8.3 One example of a social network; what others can you think of? How might you be able to make use of these social networks – both your own and those of the service user? Gartner/iStock.

Box 8.7: Vulnerability and building social networks

A study of depression amongst women on housing estates in Camberwell, UK, aimed to understand what factors lead to a woman becoming depressed. The researchers identified the following vulnerability factors:

Women

- who were at home
- had lost their mother before the age of 11
- with three children under the age of 5
- without a close confiding relationship

Women with these vulnerability factors were more likely to become depressed, particularly if they were faced by adverse life events. Working outside the home and having close networks acted as a protective factor.

(Adapted from Brown and Harris 1978)

---

class patients (Seale and Pattison 1994); yet the biggest determinant of health is poverty and inequality (Townsend et al. 1992)

If you live in one of the poorest communities you are likely to have the worst facilities – schools, hospitals, social services – and demand is usually high. This is called the inverse care law (Hart 1971). These dimensions of inequality are often best addressed by organizations closest to communities, working in partnership, and encouraging networking by service users. But, of course, not everyone feels the same about networking in this way and people use networks according to their individual circumstances and value system. McCabe et al. (1997) categorized people who use networks as:

Enthusiasts who believe that networking encourages greater local participation and innovation. Enthusiasts value networking because it overcomes the constraints of bureaucratic systems, organisational boundaries and narrow institutional policies.

Activists who view networks as a managerial approach to ensure that strategic goals are met and that initiatives are delivered in an integrated way.

Pragmatists who see networks as a necessary evil in the sense that they have to be up and running in order to secure funding from government programmes.

Opponents who are hostile to networks because they can be oppressive and imply that poor neighbourhoods can pull themselves up by their own bootstraps.

Pause Point 8.5 is designed to encourage you to think about your feelings on the process of using networks. Leaner Exercise 8.3 sets you the task of mapping your own network, considering how you might use this network if you needed care and then comparing this to someone who uses your services.

Pause Point 8.5: Your attitude to networks

What is your attitude to networks generally?
Are you an enthusiast, activist, pragmatist or opponent – or a mixture of all of these?
Can you think of one or two examples of how your attitude to networks has influenced the way you have dealt with recent life events or work?

(Adapted from Pierson 2002)

Learner Exercise 8.3: Mapping your own networks using an ecogram

Take a large piece of paper, draw a circle in the middle and place your name in it. Draw a large circle around this first circle and write in the names of your family, friends, acquaintances, social groups, clubs, organizations and agencies you have a connection with. Draw circles around each name. Think about what sort of relationships and connections you have with the various organizations, agencies, groups, families and individuals that you named.

Indicate the nature of the relationship between you and the other circles by a line linking them. Use thick lines to indicate strong connections, broken lines for weak connections. and wavy or crossed lines where there is stress associated with the connection.

Now consider that you have had a serious fall and have broken your thigh bone.
   You are going to be in hospital for several months and using crutches when you come out. How will you manage? Who will you ask for help?
Remember to think about how you would deal with your finances, your day-to-day care and housing needs.
Identify the people in your support system you feel comfortable asking for help and those you might have a more difficult relationship with if they had to help you.

Notice that there is an important difference between social networks and caring and support networks: people that you have social contact with might not want to or be willing or able to take on a caring role. Remember that it is not always about how often you see someone; it might be very important just to know they are there. Sometimes emotional support can be from someone in another country.

Now think about how this might apply to a service user that you are in contact with? Who is in their support system? Where are the gaps?

Systems theory

Ecograms are based on systems theory. These ideas originated in biology but have since been developed as a way of understanding the interactive context of social life. Systemic work has been particularly used as a way of seeing how families interact as a *system* – this is the basis for family therapy. Here we are using a systems approach to interprofessional networking. A systemic approach sees individuals not as isolated unconnected beings but as social beings, affected by and influencing others around them, the organizations with which they have contact and wider society (Payne 1997).

This acknowledgement is important. It recognizes that a child in need, a depressed mother with a young child to look after, or an older person caring for someone with dementia, affect those around them. In turn, the response of those around them affects their well-being either positively or negatively. Close family and friendship networks (when people have these) are one part of the picture. Another consists of the voluntary and community sector resources that can be drawn on to enhance social networks, building on an individual's or family's strengths. One agency in either the statutory or voluntary sector is often not enough on its own: that is why partnership working is important.

Parker and Bradley (2003) suggest that systems theory also provides a link to seeing anti-oppressive practice as challenging the oppression embedded within social structures, organizations and practices, and not simply as personal prejudice directed by one person to another. Using the theory in this way raises issues and questions like the one in the list below.

- The child in need might be of mixed heritage – does this influence the way that services respond to her? Should it?
- A mother might be a teenage parent: will this influence how the midwives, health visitors and social workers treat her? What services might she be most comfortable with?
- A person with dementia is being cared for by a lesbian couple: will this influence the service response? What kind of care home might this person be most comfortable within?

A systems approach considers the implications that social structures, the kinds of help and support provided, and access to help and support, have on the ways in which individuals, families, groups and communities operate. This can be especially useful when it's necessary to work across service junctions. People using public services meet different types of junctions in their lives, for example:

- Patients with cancer when they move from having acute care to palliative care
- Learning-disabled children reaching the age when they no longer attend school
- New mothers leaving maternity care and caring for their new infant at home.

Another example is when young people who have been in care reach adulthood. At this time the services available to support them change and this transition can be particularly difficult. Not only do the services that are provided change, but the people they meet to discuss their use of these services are different. Everyone in the team has to get to know each other and begin the process of learning about, from and with each other. It is a time when interprofessional working is essential.

The story of Casey and her support network in Case Study 8.2 demonstrates this. As you read this story, make a list of all the different services that Casey has been in contact with. Make some notes about the role of Anna, her advocate. In particular, what do you notice about Anna's relationship to Casey?

In the following list are some things that have happened while Anna has been working with Casey. Read them and make notes on how you might have reacted if you had been given professional responsibility for Casey. This is something you might be asked to do in your first job, and remember you may be of a similar age (nineteen years) to your client.

Case Study 8.2: Working with an advocate and a young adult who has been in care

Scene 1 Anna the advocate speaks. . .

I work in a detached youth work project which works with young people from aged eleven to twenty-five. I have been working with Casey for the last four years since she was nineteen – she was brought by her then boyfriend to our drop-in, she was homeless and was going to have a baby. In our project we offer intensive one-to-one support, we go with young people to meetings, to the doctor, speak on their behalf and help them to negotiate with agencies such as health, housing and social services.

Casey grew up in foster care and was living at that time in a hostel, having got into arrears and not managed to keep her flat. She wanted to keep the baby but the chaos she was living in went against her. The worker who came to assess her was not very experienced. She didn't give Casey the opportunity to go into a mother-and-baby unit for assessment; she just focused on her deficits. I wasn't experienced enough at the time to challenge this. I have learnt since then that assessments have to be positive as well as negative; they need to look at strengths as well as weaknesses, even when that is difficult.

Casey's a lovely young woman; she likes Harry Potter and has improved in her self-care enormously. We have been able to build up a relationship over four years; it is purely voluntary but she keeps coming back. Probably for the first time in her life, she has had someone who has followed all the things that have happened to her over a period of time. Before now she always had workers who had come and gone.

In this time her health has improved – she has been to the dentist (the teeth of people who have grown up in care have often been neglected), her self-care has improved, she can get money and pay rent – and her budgeting is a bit better.

At the age of twenty-one, the Social Services Leaving Care team no longer have any responsibility for young people who have been through the care system – but we carry on until they are twenty-five. She has been paying £5 a week off her debts – this is very unusual and when the housing worker praised her for doing that at a meeting she lit up.

- You been asked to visit and help make an assessment of Casey and her baby. In the car she asks you for a cigarette: how might you respond?
- The advocate is concerned that when you visited Casey you only stayed a short time. In your assessment you listed all Casey's problems and none of her strengths. She has raised this with your manager. How do you feel?
- You have been told to meet with Casey, who is homeless, to discuss her new pregnancy. You contact Anna, the advocate, to see

if she knows how to find Casey. She is reluctant to disclose this information without Casey's consent as her work has different thresholds of confidentiality from your own. How might you respond?

- Casey isn't tidying her hostel room. The room is in chaos with old food and cigarettes (you are not allowed to smoke in the building). She is in danger of being thrown out. Casey and her advocate meet with you. You learn from the advocate that Casey has made some progress and that she is grieving for her baby, who has been put up for adoption. She is very underweight. Her teeth have not been taken care of recently. What support might you offer to Casey? What role can interprofessional working play in supporting Casey at this time in her life? What do you think could be done to ease these transitions by the patchwork of agencies?

Case Study 8.2 continued

Scene 2 Anna's words sometime later

The time is coming when Casey will be too old for this project; she is withdrawing and becoming more chaotic. She has a controlling boyfriend, and is spending more time with him and becoming more distant from us. She is losing weight. I am worried about him and his friends and how vulnerable she is.

   She has never been involved in drug-taking but I wonder if he is. I wonder if she is withdrawing because she knows that we will have to stop working with her when she is twenty-five. To be honest, I have been thinking about moving on myself, but the thing that worries me most about leaving the project is leaving her.

In the scenes of Casey's story, did you notice the different roles that voluntary and statutory organizations played in her life, and how at times their priorities were different? When this happens it leads to tensions between agencies and people. Working interprofessionally helps everyone to recognize each other's strengths, understand each other's priorities and seek resolutions to any disagreements. Perhaps now is a good time to remind yourself about the key principles of interprofessional working that we set out in chapter 2. How would applying these help Casey?

Social exclusion

The sections above looked at ways of enhancing people's feelings of being included in their society and ways of increasing their access to key public sector agencies and organizations. If these measures are not in place, or if they fail to work effectively, the result is social exclusion. The quote from Pierson, below, gives a definition of

---

Box 8.8: Characteristics of social exclusion

Poverty and low income.
Lack of access to the jobs market.
Thin or non-existent social supports and networks.
The effect of the local area or neighbourhood.
Exclusion from services.

Box 8.9: Building blocks to tackling social exclusion

Maximizing income and securing basic resources.
Strengthening social supports and networks.
Working in partnership with agencies and local organizations.
Creating channels for effective participation for users, local residents and their organizations.
Focusing on whole neighbourhoods.

---

social exclusion. Note that this includes poverty but goes beyond that to encompass other factors. The characteristics of social exclusion and ways of reducing this are listed in Boxes 8.8 and 8.9. As a practitioner, you will often be working with individuals or small groups. In this chapter we are stressing the importance of their social context and some ways to help to keep this in mind. Think about this in the context of a service user you have recently worked with. How can interprofessional working and partnerships between statutory, voluntary and community organizations help them? Where is your role in this patchwork of people and service settings?

> Social exclusion is a process that deprives individuals and families, groups and neighbourhoods of the resources required for participation in the social economic and political activity of society as a whole. This process is primarily a consequence of poverty and low income but other factors such as discrimination, low educational attainment and depleted living environments also underpin it. Through this process people are cut off for a significant period in their lives from institutions and services, social networks and developmental opportunities that the great majority of a society enjoys.
> (Pierson 2002, p. 7)

Another way of looking at social exclusion is to see it as a form of alienation from society. Keating (1998) identified five levels of alienation in the context of the French colonization of Algeria (Box

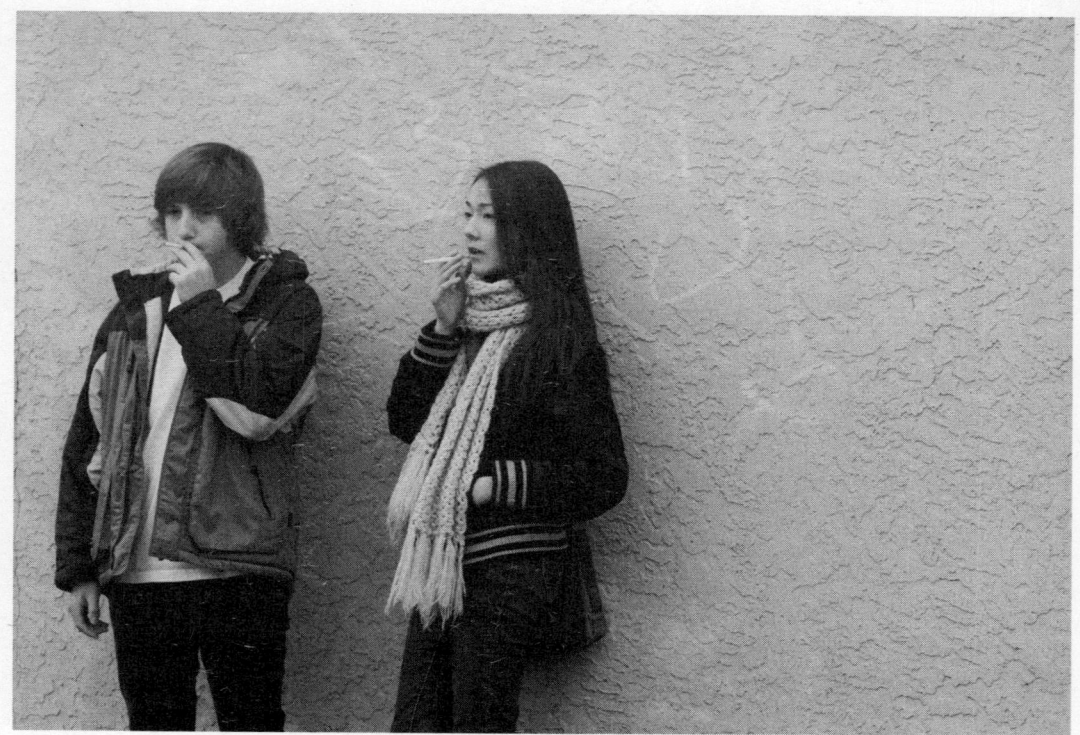

Photo 8.4 It is important that nobody is excluded from service provision – for example, some young people may appear to refuse help or might be judged on their behaviour (such as smoking, irresponsible drinking or unprotected sex) and thus excluded from the full support of practitioners. Christian Stewart/iStock.

Box 8.10: Levels of alienation

The first level is alienation from the self – for example having little sense of self, of self esteem, poor self care, poor hygiene, not eating.

The second level is alienation from significant others – partner, close friends, family.

The third level is alienation from your peer group, friends and networks.

The fourth level is alienation from your own cultural norms and traditions and relates to colonisation of a less powerful group by a dominant group.

The fifth is alienation from society including jobs, housing and employment.

(Keating 1998)

8.10). This might be a helpful tool to use with someone you are working with. One way of representing this is to place the service user at the centre with concentric circles around them to indicate the different levels.

Pause Point 8.6: Casey and the framework of alienation

Think about what you know of Casey, using the framework in Box 8.8.

Can you see themes emerging?

How can this help you gain a picture of what social exclusion means in her situation, and the range of services and interventions that can assist Casey?

Social inclusion and mental health

Mental distress is one of the most contested areas of health and social care, and mental illness carries a considerable stigma (Tew 2005). Mainstream mental health services are in the process of adopting a recovery approach. This means looking at what can be done to enhance recovery overall rather than focusing all attention on alleviating symptoms. In some places, mental health services work with and help to fund daycare services, counselling, befriending, complementary therapies, advice work and physical well-being services. All of these have been shown to enhance service users' lives and respond to their wishes. Partnership between statutory and voluntary agencies in mental health services is often seen as a promising way forward, but also highlights issues of clinical and personal responsibility, confidentiality and fairness (Tait and Shah 2007). It can also involve sharing information about services users across agency and professional boundaries. In chapter 9 we look at the challenges of this in detail for a number of different situations.

Many users of the mental health services also have children. A family in this situation might come to the attention of education, social and health statutory services. Parrott et al. (2008) summarize current knowledge about the relationship between stress and resilience factors for parents with mental health problems and their children: one aspect their work looks at is the role of practical and emotional social support and the role of different agencies.

One problem often faced by mental health service users is the feeling of isolation from their social networks. Learner Exercise 8.4 focuses on Jack, who has mental health problems, and the alienation framework in Box 8.8. It is designed so that you can test how the theoretical model can be helpful in your practice. Inviting members of your interprofessional team to do the exercise with you and then comparing notes should give you all an insight into the different perspectives that practitioners from different work settings bring to the service offered to one client.

As we all know from our personal and practice experience, isolation is not experienced only by people with mental health problems. If you are unlikely to meet someone like Jack in your work setting, you can do Learner Exercise 8.4 with someone else in mind – someone who uses your services and might feel similarly isolated.

Learner Exercise 8.5: Helping Jack feel less isolated

Jack is in his early sixties. His wife died some years ago. He has recently been discharged from psychiatric hospital after being there for six months. He has one son but has no contact with him because his son believes Jack to have been abusive, which he denies. Jack had no visitors during his stay in hospital but got on well socially with most staff and patients. When he was in hospital he attended the local church and local pub, alone or with other patients. He drinks regularly but moderately. He is able to cook and look after himself, so he has been discharged home to his flat. Jack self-medicates plus receives a fortnightly injection. He uses the bus, but lives in a fairly remote village with infrequent buses and will be visited at home occasionally by the care coordinator.

   You are asked to go and visit Jack to help with his isolation.

What kinds of resources might you use for this work?

How can you use the five levels of alienation framework to assess what kinds of support you think he needs?

Assess whether the framework was useful to you in identifying what might help Jack.

Your focus could be on a newly bereaved wife, a first-time single mother or a young man involved in a road traffic accident whose recent job move means he is living a very long way from friends and family.

Public participation and consultation

When you are working interprofessionally, it is good to be clear about what level of participation you are hoping for from the voluntary and community sectors, and what level is feasible within your context. Pierson (2002, p. 58) writes that:

> Whilst practitioners may be individually committed to maximum levels of user participation, they will often find legal obligations, agency policies and user expectations all constrain participation.

It can be helpful to understand levels of participation for service users in your setting by using a model of the range of different levels of participation. So we have included Arnstein's (1969) ladder of citizen participation (table 8.1) to enable you to compare and contrast the reality with theory. The ladder maps the different gradations of what 'participation' can mean. Higher levels denote citizens having more power and control, middle levels of the ladder denote participation that is more token, and the lowest levels denote being *done to*, rather than being able to participate actively in decision-making

Table 8.1 Ladder of citizen participation

Degrees of citizen power	Citizen Control
	Delegated power
Degrees of tokenism	Partnership
	Placation
	Consultation
Degrees of non participation	Informing
	Therapy
	Manipulation

Source: Arnstein 1969

about initiatives or services by service users, citizens, community or voluntary organizations. It's always good to see how something works in terms of your own experiences, so Pause Point 8.7 asks you to apply the ladder to your experience as a student.

Pause Point 8.7: Assessing levels of consultation and participation

Have you been consulted recently as a student about anything?
Where do you think that consultation sits on the ladder of citizen participation?
Has the outcome of the consultation changed any of the decisions that were made?

To conclude

In this chapter we explored the value and range of the contribution made by the voluntary and community sectors to effective interprofessional practice. We also looked at how private organizations are involved with providing services for well-being, health and to meet the daily living needs of service users.

Two key contributions of the voluntary and community sectors are: the importance of experience and having *been there*; and a *strengths* approach, which focuses on people's abilities, active involvements, networks and own coping strategies, rather than their deficits. The private sector will provide more services to meet social and health-care needs in the twenty-first century, alongside those provided by the statutory sector. We identified strategies for finding out about the range of resources that are available to all service users and how you might signpost people to these. We hope that you now feel able to use the concepts of networking and social inclusion in your interprofessional practice.

Part III

Drawing Together the Threads

In Part II we examined the multiple and overlapping frameworks that make up the reality of interprofessional practice. How and when you work with users of services, carers, and the type and number of practitioner colleagues in the interprofessional team, will depend on your particular area of work. It will vary from time to time; changes in policy and practice will have their influence and so will your career moves. As you read in the last chapter the voluntary, community and private sectors have an increasingly important role in the delivery of effective public services. Your work may take you into one of these directly as a worker or as a team member with people from those sectors. You may extend your use of services; you may find out what it's like to be a carer.

Whatever area you work in, more and more emphasis is placed on the importance and challenges of information sharing between practitioners about the user of their services. We also acknowledge that our readers will continue their lives and careers in rewarding jobs that recognize the advantage of their ability to be interprofessional.

In Part III we look at these two issues as fundamental to the practice and working lives of all practitioners. First we examine the critical issue of information sharing; then we discuss the continuation and elaboration of working life for interprofessional practitioners.

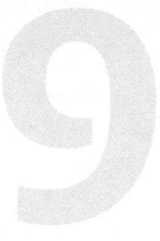

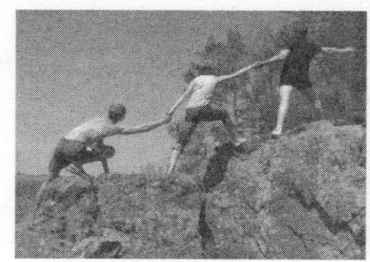

9

Sharing Information: The Continuing Challenge

My whole life is waiting for the questions to which I have prepared answers.

Tom Stoppard

What you will read in this chapter

We now return to an issue that has been a thread in many other chapters: to the continuing challenge for the interprofessional team of sharing information. Inescapably, this is linked with how practitioners, service users and carers communicate with each other, although, as we show, poor communication is but one factor in a number of barriers to good practice in information sharing.

The role of information

Divorced from human action, information is incapable of doing anything, simply because it is inanimate. It is what you do with information that gives it value and helps or hinders other people's work.

Practitioners gather information to guide decision-making and subsequent intervention. It is an ongoing process of gathering, analysing, deciding, acting and returning to gathering information to enable review and, if appropriate, the formulation of new plans. Inevitably, this cycle will be punctuated by periods of waiting, but we should take care that these do not become excessive.

As no practitioner works in complete isolation, it is necessary for all of us at some time to share information. The myriad of ways in which this can occur adds to the richness and complexity of professional practice. It also has a profound effect on the quality of care. Doing Learner Exercise 9.1 should help you relate this to your practice and the people you work with.

Learner Exercise 9.1: Information sharing – creating a real picture

Think about a particular service user or patient or pupil you have worked with: the task now is to create a simple picture of all the colleagues you have needed to share information with in the course of that work. Using a particular colour pen, draw this as a 'spider graph' or 'mind map', i.e., put yourself in the middle and draw all the people and connections you have had to make. Complete this by putting in arrows that show the direction of information flow.

Taking the same drawing and using a pen of a different colour, circle your service user/patient/pupil and add people you think they will have had to contact as part of the process of having their needs met – for example, in their family, social and work networks. Again show the information-flow pathways.

Finally, using yet another colour pen, consider the connections from the perspective of one of the other practitioners on your map. You might like to ask someone from the practice group or the work setting you have chosen to comment on the result of this addition.

Now consider:

- The implications of the patterns and complexity of what you have drawn
- How best to be mindful about communicating in these types of situations.

For much of our working lives information is shared according to well-established procedures, in a well-structured, well-targeted and uncontroversial manner. This may sustain effective oversight of service users' needs, coordinated input from relevant practitioners, successful outcomes and ongoing goodwill. Sometimes things are not that straightforward. We continue by examining some of the challenges associated with information sharing in professional, interprofessional and inter-agency practice.

Before you read on, quickly brainstorm some of your ideas about sharing information so that you get a clearer view of what guides your thinking and behaviour now. Pause Point 9.1 has some questions to stimulate your thinking.

Your answers to the questions in Pause Point 9.1 probably contained elements of *well, it depends upon. . .*, followed by a list of reasons. If you worked on the activity in a small group it is very likely that people had different perspectives, even if that group was from a single profession and all at the same stage in terms of education or careers. The more diverse the group, the more you may have learnt about different perspectives.

In the following sections we examine aspects of information sharing that may well impinge on your working life. Some will be illustrated with examples from reports into high-profile cases of tragedies following failures in care. These bring the issues into sharp relief. But the less dramatic, lower-level daily manifestations of the

Pause Point 9.1: Criteria for sharing information

In general, do you think your information about the history, current context, needs and wishes of any of your clients/patients/service users should be shared with other relevant practitioners on the basis of:

- The minimum they need to know to answer your questions
- As fully as possible, including things which are tentative or matters of opinion rather than verifiable facts
- Only as required by law
- As much as you can manage, given that you are always overworked
- In a manner negotiated with the service user
- According to guidelines provided by your professional body
- According to guidelines provided by your employer
- In line with an internal sense of red flags (warnings) that you have developed through experience, learning and reflection to inform your professional judgement
- In a way that fits in with the culture around you?

Learner Exercise 9.2: Information sharing – knowledge, skills and judgement

Jot down some notes quickly to capture key things from your thinking or discussions on the following questions:

- What sort of skills and knowledge do you need to share information appropriately and effectively with other practitioners or other agencies/organizations?
- What sort of professional judgements will you have to make?
- What sorts of attitudes or values influence your judgements?

same processes are just as important: possibly more so because of their higher frequency.

The aspects of information sharing that we discuss are:

- The quantity, type and timeliness of information shared
- Legal and regulatory frameworks
- Different thresholds for sharing or withholding information
- Many knew but found it too difficult to speak out
- Joining-up the dots.

All aspects of sharing information require us to know what to share and how to share it, and we all have certain attitudes that shape our judgements about who with and when to share information. This probably sounds very familiar to you! So before we set down our thinking on the aspects listed above, try doing Learner Exercise 9.2.

This is a *before and after* type of learning activity; either do it alone or in a small group. Return to it after studying the rest of the chapter and possibly some of the additional resources that we highlight. In this way, you will be able to see how your thinking and understanding have developed through your study of information sharing in this book.

The quantity, type and timeliness of information shared

We began our discussion by looking at issues that arise when information is shared as practitioners make referrals to other practitioners and services for tests, assessment, an additional opinion, therapeutic input, practical assistance and so on. It may be helpful for you to glance back at what we wrote about referral as a key part of interprofessional collaboration: you will find this in chapter 5. A number of key themes began to emerge there that we will draw out a little further here.

A key question when making a referral is about how much information should be shared. One of the challenges in this situation is that our choices about this rely on our professional judgement. We build up and refine our professional judgement throughout our working lives – at least we will refine our professional judgement if we continue to reflect on our professional practice (see chapter 5), otherwise our professional judgement may become outdated and ineffective.

Nevertheless some key principles can be elaborated. For example, if you provide too much information you may exhaust people's attention and they may miss vital parts. Another risk is that they may become distracted by something that is not central to your concern or request, and omit work that you would like them to complete. Both these risks can be mitigated by providing structure within the information that you share. This helps the recipients to identify key features and the nature of the action or opinion that you are requesting. This is why forms and templates have evolved for transmitting written information in paper-based and electronic systems. To some extent, evolved conventions in verbal communication within areas of professional practice (e.g., case reviews, handover and ward rounds) also serve to provide a structure that highlights key features of information that is shared.

Returning to the question of how much information should be shared, too little can prove just as difficult as too much. The recipients may not have sufficient information to make a decision or to appreciate the degree of need. At best this will cause delays while additional information is sought. Delays can be damaging: people deteriorate; sometimes the changes are irreversible. Options may become more limited and the ultimate burden of care may

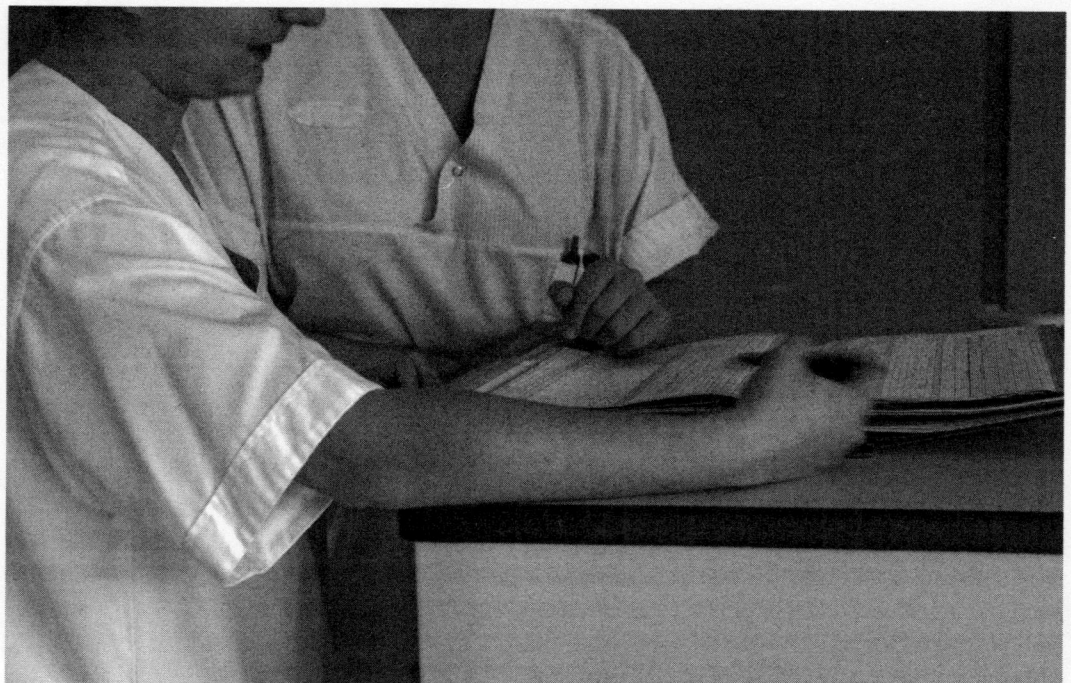

Photo 9.1 Sharing information may seem simple; however, you need to be very aware of what messages you are sending to a colleague to whom you refer a patient or client, and make sure that you present the necessary information objectively and clearly. Dr Heinz Linke/iStock

increase unnecessarily. At worse, too little information could lead to a need being overlooked and no provision made. It is possible that this would continue unnoticed until a crisis or another form of deterioration prompted reassessment.

Effective information sharing is aided by focusing on the needs and reasonable responses of those who receive information from you. We have already mentioned quantity and structure as important features of effective communication. In the opening chapter we wrote about how the unthinking use of jargon and acronyms creates a gap in understanding between people in the interprofessional team. Being a skilled communicator is essential to being interprofessional. So it is also important to think about the words, abbreviations and symbols you use. Will the recipients be familiar with these and interpret them the same way as you do? It is helpful to remember that professions and organizations develop terms and phrases that have specific meanings in specific contexts. Divorced from their context or viewed from a different area of practice, these ways of saying things may be impenetrable or, perhaps more dangerous, appear comprehensible but get ascribed a somewhat different meaning.

This is not limited to technical language. Think about the everyday term 'satisfactory'. Depending upon context, this may mean absolutely fine and everyone is happy; or it might mean not very good, key people are not content but things are not quite bad enough to be labelled 'poor'.

One way of looking at the way information moves around an organization or a group of organizations collaborating with each other is to imagine the content as water flowing in a river. There has to be a source of the information (and sometimes there are multiple sources), a route and an eventual destination. Instead of the sea or a lake, in our case the destination is the person who needs the information you are sending. Learner Exercise 9.3 asks you to look at the key points in the information flows related to your work, and to examine what works and what doesn't work so well.

Learner Exercise 9.3: Examining information flows

For your own area of practice think about how information is transmitted and received: for example, talking face to face or by telephone, written within patient notes, within referrals or requests to other practitioners or services, within case reviews or audit records.

What are the strengths and weaknesses in information sharing in your area of practice?
Are there blocks in the way of the information flow? If so, what causes them?
Do some information flows work better in some respects than in others?
Is it easier for information to flow in some circumstances than others?
What can be learnt from any variation that you have detected?
What is worth promoting elsewhere as good practice?
What are the main sources of frustration, delay or miscommunication?
What practical steps might be taken to mitigate the problems you have identified?

Keeping a focus on the needs and reasonable reactions of the recipient can help to check that the information we share is sufficiently complete for purpose and that, so far as is possible, its presentation avoids error or ambiguity. If inaccurate information is shared, inaccurate decisions will be made. If ambiguous information is shared, we cannot be sure what will happen.

The information contained in our messages to colleagues about service users/clients/patients is of different types. There are definite facts, for example, results of blood tests, and there are professional judgements based on our expertise and experience. Practitioners also use terms and phrases to describe the context surrounding the person in the communication to help colleagues' understanding of that person's situation. Some examples of this are listed in Box 9.1.

Looked at in one way, appropriate contextual information is important in helping to illuminate the significance of factual observations, providing nuanced diagnoses, promoting informed

Box 9.1: Examples of contextual information

'recently widowed'; 'poor-quality housing'; 'suspect domestic violence'; 'caring for terminally ill partner'; 'neighbours reported concerns'; 'single parent – child has leaning disabilities'; 'chaotic lifestyle'; 'housebound'; 'interested in trying complementary therapies'; 'alcoholic'; 'unplanned pregnancy'; 'recently released from prison'; 'determined to return to work'; 'uses interpreter'; or 'intermittent drug use'.

decisions and aiding the provision of user-focused care. On the other hand, incorrect information may be destructive or reinforce negative stereotypes and limit the range of options offered to the service user. Professional judgement and knowledge of others' roles and information needs are required to decide what information the recipient needs and what additional information would be helpful. It is always possible that something that appears insignificant to you is very important for another in the web of practitioners and organizations contributing to care.

Any checking process should also consider whether we are sharing information with the correct people: those appropriately placed to help our service user/client/patient. Sharing information with people who are in no position to contribute to the web of care that a particular person requires wastes time and possibly other resources. It also causes frustration and might reduce goodwill or trust. In certain circumstances it may constitute an inappropriate breech of confidentiality. Learner Exercise 9.4 gives you the opportunity to see how this applies in your practice setting.

While not wishing to overburden colleagues and systems, it is important to engage in periodic updating. This allows decisions and

Learner Exercise 9.4: Sharing contextual information

Think about your own area of professional practice.

What kinds of contextual information are you likely to share (send and receive) with other practitioners and other organizations?
Consider the disclosure of pre-existing conditions, demographic information or statements like those in Box 9.1.
What influence does such information have on the service you provide?
What would be the likely impact if any of this contextual information was incorrect or misunderstood?

If possible discuss the perspective you have from your area of practice with somebody from a different area of practice.

plans to be reviewed in the light of changes and new information. It also provides an opportunity to detect and correct errors or misunderstandings. Many areas of practice have well-developed mechanisms for periodic updating: team meetings, case conferences and reviews, ward rounds, handover briefings and so on. If your practice area lacks well-developed updating mechanisms to which all relevant people contribute information and analyses, you will have greater individual responsibility to update and review. This should be done sufficiently often to detect changes that will influence your practice.

Legal and regulatory frameworks

Legal and regulatory frameworks affect the way information is stored and shared. This is not only due to what these laws and regulations require and prohibit, but also due to practitioners' (sometimes inaccurate) perceptions of what is required and what is prohibited. Indeed, if practitioners are not sure what they can or should share, a culture may develop in which it is seen to be *safest* to share very little. This begs the question *safest for whom*? Service users, the wider public, practitioners or organizations that provide services? A degree of uncertainty is understandable; multiple sources and layers of regulation do exist and have led to the perception of regulation as an early twenty-first-century growth industry.

Laws vary from country to country, even between the four countries forming the United Kingdom. In addition, different levels of legislature may coexist. For example, in Europe, European law coexists (or competes) with national law; and in many countries around the globe administrative units such as states, provinces or homelands have legislative and regulatory powers that must coexist with national legislation and regulation.

As we might expect, the law is largely silent with respect to interprofessional and inter-agency collaboration. Normally this would be an inappropriate level of detail for legislative attention. An exception in England is the Children Act (2004). This imposes upon practitioners who work with children a duty to cooperate to improve well-being (Section 10) and to safeguard and promote the welfare of children (Section 11). You will recall that we referred to this Act in chapter 4. Why do you think this Act imposes these duties on practitioners?

Some legislation for other purposes does have an impact on collaborative practice. For example, the Data Protection Act (1998) regulates the electronic storage of personal information: the nature of what is kept and for how long; maintaining confidentiality when appropriate and disclosing certain information when appropriate. In this way, legislation affects how practitioners and organizations create and store records for their clients and about their services. From time to time, concerns about the legality of keeping or sharing certain information are cited as reasons for destroying or withholding information that may help other practitioners or agencies fulfil their roles. Mostly these concerns are unfounded, based on limited understanding of the legislation and its objectives. Less often, the curbing of collaboration is deemed an acceptable price for safeguards against unfettered linking of information with the consequent loss of privacy and risk of errors proliferating.

The Human Rights Act (1998) is another area that places certain limits on information sharing. Fears of contravening this poorly understood (and often misquoted) legislation may lead to unnecessary caution in sharing information. In the UK, the state has devolved some of its power to recognized professional bodies, allowing these to regulate membership of the profession in a number of ways. Professional bodies publish rules and guidelines to inform practitioners and the public. Interprofessional collaboration for the benefit of service users is normally encouraged. Information sharing may be addressed in a number of ways – for example, through setting out expectations in relation to maintaining confidentiality in most circumstances *and* identifying duties to disclose information in certain circumstances: particularly when significant harm is thought likely. Leaner Exercise 9.5 encourages you to find out more about this for your profession and one other profession, and to consider the impact on your practice of your findings.

Learner Exercise 9.5: Examining the rules and guidelines on information sharing

Assess how much you already know about laws, regulations, policies and guidelines for information sharing for your profession?

Look up your own profession's website to find their rules and guidance in relation to information sharing and also interprofessional collaboration or inter-agency working.

Now try this for a profession with which you expect to work closely.

Are their rules and guidance on information sharing and interprofessional or inter-agency collaboration essentially the same as for your own profession?

How significant are the differences you find?

How might these differences impact on your interprofessional practice?

Different workplaces also have different guidelines and procedures for sharing information. This arises because of differences in historical context and organizational function; and variation in the focus of activities and local cultures. When you move between workplaces, or work with colleagues from different workplaces, it is wise not to assume that everyone shares a common set of principles and rules governing the way that they share information to support collaborative practice.

Different thresholds for sharing or withholding information

The different thresholds for sharing or withholding information that we outlined above are all based on reasonable judgements about what practitioners should do. In reality and in everyday work the standards they set may not be attained by everyone. This occurs for a wide range of reasons and the consequences can be unpredictable.

Sometimes there is selfishness, obstructive behaviour or thoughtlessness that prevents or slows the sharing of information, creating ill-will and quite possibly causing gaps in care. Sometimes professional judgements to withhold information are based on a longer-term view of how best to help certain service users. Of course, the appropriateness of each such professional judgement lies predominantly in the eye of the beholder. We can only confirm such decisions as good or bad with the benefit of hindsight. In Case Study 9.1 we tell the story of two practitioners, a community worker and a midwife, who are both trying to do their best for Gemma, their client. After reading the scenario, take a few minutes to reflect on the questions in Pause Point 9.2.

Case Study 9.1: Gemma

Lena is a community worker. Over the past few months she has carefully established a relationship with Gemma, a young woman who lives in difficult circumstances. She has a controlling and sometimes violent partner, very limited social networks and now an unplanned pregnancy. Lena is approached by Sunita, a midwife, who knows that Gemma has moved on from the address she supplied at her booking appointment, but now Sunita cannot find her. Sunita has some test results to discuss with Gemma and phones Lena to ask for her new address. In the call, Sunita gives no clue to Lena about the seriousness or urgency of her need to contact Gemma. Although she realizes that Gemma should see a midwife, Lena decides that giving the new address may be perceived as a large breach of trust by her client. Lena fears that this might mean Gemma will withdraw from contact with her and may well refuse to see the midwife again anyway. Building sufficient trust to work productively with this young woman was slow with frequent setbacks, but Lena is pleased that recently it has been working well. Gemma still feels let down by past contacts with statutory health and social care services, but is gaining in confidence through engagement with activities available through the charity that employs Lena. She is looking after herself better, making more active and considered decisions, and beginning to carry more of these decisions through. Lena decides she must check with Gemma before disclosing her new address.

On this occasion, Lena's threshold for sharing information is higher than Sunita had hoped for and she takes a very dim view of this, frustrated at the inevitable delay. She even goes as far as to say that Lena has no right to be obstructive, that her attitude is unprofessional and she is not qualified to make these decisions. The call ends and the two staff are very unhappy with one another. Lena resolves to contact the young woman as soon as possible and try to help her to re-establish contact with antenatal services.

Pause Point 9.2: A reflection on Case Study 9.1

Who is right in this situation described in Case Study 9.1?

How much is your view coloured by the range of outcomes that you perceive? How much is it coloured by your profession's view of the nature of good care?

Try to think of four different endings for Case Study 9.1 (work with others if you run out of ideas).

One other variation in information-sharing thresholds happens at the boundary of the immediate work team and other more distant staff or teams. Members of the immediate work team may share information freely and effectively, but set higher thresholds before sharing information with others outside this team, even though they are involved in the care of the same client/patient or service user. When we make these distinctions, we should examine the rationale for the differences and the extent to which they help or hinder the collaborative effort to do the best and most appropriate things possible within finite resources. This can often happen in inter-agency working and at the transition points of a client/patient/service user's journey, as we discussed in chapters 4 and 8.

Many knew but it was too difficult to say

In this section we draw on the Report of the Bristol Royal Infirmary Inquiry (Kennedy et al. 2001) into higher than expected deaths following children's heart surgery in the period 1984–95. This is a vivid example of a situation in which several factors combined to make it difficult for a range of practitioners with concerns to voice them. Further, when concerns were voiced it was difficult for these to be heard and acted upon effectively. At the Bristol Royal Infirmary the death rates for babies undergoing heart surgery was twice that of other hospitals. The public inquiry into this found there was sufficient data and professional knowledge available to enable much earlier action to remedy problems, as the quote in Box 9.2 confirms. But the dominant professional culture discouraged information sharing, with the result that the problems continued for years.

The paragraph given in Box 9.2 goes on to note that very limited amounts of information were shared with families and the general

> **Box 9.2: A key finding of Kennedy et al. (2001)**
>
> Bristol was awash with data. There was enough information from the late 1980s onwards to cause questions about mortality rates to be raised both in Bristol and elsewhere had the mindset to do so existed.
>
> (Report summary, paragraph 18: openness)

public. This meant that the public had to rely on health-care practitioners and their employers to share and scrutinize information in order for problems to be detected and rectified, and patients protected.

Chapters 11 and 12 of the Report (Kennedy et al. 2001) examine expression of concerns by individuals and reactions to the concerns raised. It is clear that a wide range of people had concerns, including managers, anaesthetists, cardiologists, surgeons, a pathologist, a radiographer and nurses. Audit data persistently showed excess mortality. This was explained in terms of low volumes and the complex case mix, and was difficult to refute in the short term. These explanations were accepted in preference to closer scrutiny of the quality of care.

Audit data can be difficult to collect and aggregate. This renders it relatively easy to discredit if discussions focus on the detail of the data, rather than on general messages such as 'it looks like there may be a problem here which needs full and open discussion'. Furthermore the organizational and professional seniority and power of the surgeons at the centre of the concerns made it difficult for people to speak out, and diminished the chances of their perceptions being treated as accurate. Consequently people's concerns were often raised indirectly, and were easily deflected or simply overlooked, despite the ingenious nature of some attempts at exposure. These included publishing an academic paper and articles in a widely read satirical magazine; sharing audit data with academic colleagues from the local university and handing audit data to a senior UK Department of Health official; and the refusal of two nurses to participate when the problematic procedure was undertaken. All this occurred alongside more conventional attempts from a number of people to discuss concerns among colleagues with a view to harnessing concern into effective action. For too long, it proved too difficult to achieve sufficiently widespread consensus that there were problems, without which there could be no desire or plans for effective corrective action. By now you are probably wondering just why it took so long.

The problems with raising and acknowledging concerns were largely cultural. People were fearful of challenging senior surgeons. The status of the clinical unit as a regional supra centre and an academic centre created expectations that work would be conducted at the leading edge of the discipline. Problems were also masked by developments that spanned more than a decade. These included

Pause Point 9.3: Voices, concerns and criticism

- In your area of practice are there situations in which it is difficult to voice opinions or raise concerns and be heard?
- What kind of knowledge would you need to raise concerns?
- If you wanted to say something that you thought might not be welcomed, how would you prepare?
- How can you make it easier for people to say things to you that might feel like criticism?

retirements, plans for recruitment of an experienced surgeon from a leading centre elsewhere, and long-running plans to physically consolidate children's services in a new hospital. For a long time it was too easy to argue that past or current problems were on the road to resolution through planned change.

The magnitude and duration of problems uncovered by the Bristol Royal Infirmary Inquiry make it relatively easy to feel that it is extreme and would never happen where you work. After all, lessons have been learnt and received widespread publicity. But we encourage you to use Pause Point 9.3 to reflect for a moment about less vivid examples in places where you are likely to work. It is also worth noting that problems in speaking out and being heard are also central to reports from contrasting areas of care. We go on to discuss another example involving psychiatric care.

The UK Department of Heath ordered an independent inquiry into the way that concerns raised by patients of two consultant psychiatrists (William Kerr and Michael Haslam) had been dealt with (DoH 2005b). In 2003 Michael Haslam was convicted of four charges of indecent assault on three patients and jailed for three years; William Kerr was convicted (in his absence) on one count of indecent assault. The inquiry heard testimony from more than sixty people that the two doctors had sexually assaulted patients over a twenty-year period. Many of the women had complained to their family doctors and to nurses. Concerns had also been raised with local solicitors and the police. The inquiry posed three central questions about why complaints and concerns did not lead to investigation and action (Box 9.3). It concluded that, alongside management failure, poor record-keeping and a culture in which consultants were extremely powerful, failed communication had been crucial. Some people ignored warning signs; some people chose to remain silent when, with the benefit of hindsight, the inquiry judged they should have spoken out; and others tried to speak out but were not heard.

Box 9.4 contains part of an account from a former patient, reflecting upon the failed communication and a little of its impact on those who were abused.

Box 9.3: Central questions in the Kerr/Haslem Inquiry

- How could it be that the voices of the patients and former patients of William Kerr and Michael Haslem were not heard?
- Why were so many opportunities to respond and investigate missed?
- How could it happen that abuse of patients, evidenced by the convictions of William Kerr and Michael Haslem, went undetected for so long?'

(DoH 2005b, executive summary, para 2)

Box 9.4: A comment on attitudes and behaviour in response to complaints

During the inquiry many doctors, nurses and former hospital managers gave their evidence and in many cases excuses as to why even though they admitted they were aware of a 'problem' they did nothing. The words 'I cannot recall' or 'have no recollection' must have been the most widely repeated of all throughout the hearings. There were some nurses and doctors who had tried to alert those in authority but got nowhere. I think we all felt some sympathy for those who had tried to do something but there was a lot of anger towards those who either would not, or could not or did not do anything . . .

(Haq 2006)

The Kerr/Haslam Inquiry found an 'absence of multidisciplinary working' and 'Over-rigid interpretation, or even misinterpretation, of the legal position pertaining to the requirement for patient confidentiality – such that it overrode patient safety' (DoH 2005b executive summary, p. 13). Both these findings were seen as barriers to investigating and acting upon patients' complaints. Both signal the need for attention to enhancing collaboration and improving information-sharing practice (as discussed throughout this book). Note also that two of the recommendations of the Kerr/Haslam Inquiry were the need for better training for staff in complaint handling and independent advocacy for patients. Take a moment to reflect on your learning needs about complaint handling and to check if you know about patient advocacy arrangements in your work setting.

Joining up the dots

Most people will have first-hand experience of the children's activity books in which numbered dots must be joined in sequence before a picture is revealed. The process of interprofessional and inter-agency teams sharing information effectively can be the same. In this section

Box 9.5: A failure to protect

It is deeply disturbing that during the days and months following her initial contact with Ealing Housing Department's Homeless Persons' Unit, Victoria was known to no less than two further housing authorities, four social services departments, two child protection teams of the Metropolitan Police Service, a specialist centre managed by the NSPCC, and she was admitted to two different hospitals because of suspected deliberate harm. The dreadful reality was that these services knew little or nothing more about Victoria at the end of the process than they did when she was first referred to Ealing Social Services by the Homeless Persons' Unit in April 1999.[1] The final irony was that Haringey Social Services formally closed Victoria's case on the very day she died. The extent of the failure to protect Victoria was lamentable.

[1] Victoria died on 25 Feb 2000.

(Laming 2003, paragraph 1.16)

we look at some aspects of the report into the probably preventable death of Victoria Climbié (Laming 2003). Joining up the dots was not the only important issue in this case. Lord Laming identified 'widespread organizational malaise' (paragraph 1.21) as the principal cause of failure to protect Victoria. The two people to whom Victoria's care was entrusted were convicted of her murder: criminal behaviour that included months of cruelty. It was a case well beyond the experience of the people who had contact with Victoria. Nevertheless, failure to join up the dots was also significant, as the quote in Box 9.5 shows.

One fundamental problem in this case was that as Victoria moved from agency to agency, and location to location, the front-line housing and social work staff, health practitioners, police officers, voluntary sector staff and volunteers, and members of the public who encountered Victoria or her case tended to view their contact in isolation. They interpreted what they learnt without seeing the extent of the wider pattern of her deteriorating health and increasing abuse. Record systems did not facilitate easy linking of all these separate contacts, even within different parts of the health service.

Front-line staff and their managers failed to investigate and review Victoria's case sufficiently diligently to link together several reports of suspected deliberate harm. They did not adequately appreciate her deteriorating well-being. Several people who suspected deliberate harm did little to follow through their concerns. Even those who documented their concerns and passed this information to others sometimes did so ambiguously or ambivalently. Those who received ambiguous information seem not to have sought clarification. There were more than a dozen 'dots', and joining even a few of these would probably have galvanized people into removing Victoria to a safe place and keeping her away from harm.

As we wrote in chapter 4, this case led to the *Every Child Matters: Change for Children* (<www.everychildmatters.co.uk>) agenda in England. It is worth repeating again that this promotes the importance of well-functioning multi-agency panels and teams, integrated services and a lead professional role. It provides a common assessment framework for practitioners to use and guidance on information sharing. Workforce reform and training needs are addressed; and the programme is pushing towards a unified record for each child to increase the probability of *joining the dots* in time to help and protect children in need. Legislation has been changed to facilitate such a record (Children Act 2004).

It is argued that the later legislation is consistent with the Human Rights Act (1998) (remember how that featured in our framework for the development of service-user participation in chapter 6) and the Data Protection Act (1998). It seeks to safeguard the rights of children, young people and families to see information relating to themselves and have errors corrected. Doing Learner Exercise 9.6 should help you to identify some resources about information sharing, and to develop an understanding of good practice, when you need to share information with colleagues in the interprofessional team.

Failure to join dots is a depressingly frequent occurrence. Many families will be able to tell stories of less dramatic failures to connect information into a meaningful picture, delaying or preventing the provision of appropriate care and support. In more serious cases the failure leads to a fatality, as the information in Box 9.6 confirms.

Learner Exercise 9.6: Resources and gaining insight into information-sharing practices

Look at the information-sharing section of the Every Child Matters website: <www.everychildmatters.co.uk/deliveringservices/informationsharing>.

Even if you don't work with children, the Common Assessment Framework for Children and Young People: Practitioners' Guide (Children's Workforce Development Council 2007) provides helpful clarification on the nature of confidentiality, relevant aspects of consent and the concept of proportionality. It sets out clear guidance on issues to consider when sharing information and there is a useful glossary.

It is also worth looking at some of the case studies that illustrate how more effective information sharing can be achieved and linked to providing better services (Department for Children, Schools and Families 2005)

Can you find similar resources for your own area of practice?
Try to work in a small group and compare your findings with those of others.

Box 9.6: Another failure to protect

Christopher Clunis killed Jonathan Zito on a platform at Finsbury Park underground station, North London, in 1992. Staff from a number of agencies, the police, doctors, psychiatric nurses and social workers, failed to correctly assess the risk of violence. None of them *joined up the dots* despite the fact that eight days before the attack Christopher had been found wandering around the streets with a screwdriver and a breadknife, attacking people.

The inquiry into Jonathan's death found that the agencies did not communicate well with each other and practitioners within agencies did not communicate well with each other. There was little overall effort made to obtain a complete record of Christopher's history over time and *join up the dots* when he presented to individual services in a particular area, or to communicate and keep in touch with his family.

There were other issues that contributed to Jonathan Zito's death. These included resource problems within the services involved, Christopher moving to different areas and stopping taking his medication. But a lack of *joining up of the dots* and not carrying out a proper risk assessment were also key contributing factors in this failure to protect.

(Adapted from Ritchie et al. 1994)

The Report of the Confidential Inquiry into Homicides and Suicides by Mentally Ill People (Royal College of Psychiatrists 1996) identified that failures of communication between practitioners, and between practitioners and carers/families, were factors that contributed to otherwise preventable deaths by people with mental illness. Its key recommendations were the need for support for the development of genuine multidisciplinary teams, and developing better systems for communication between practitioners and between practitioners and families. It is important to note that the vast majority of people with mental illness are not violent to others, although their risk of suicide is higher. Homicide committed by people with mental health problems is rare despite media reports to the contrary. However, when there is this rare risk, as the report cited above shows, *joining up the dots* has an important role in reducing this to as low a risk as is humanly possible. Being prepared for the challenges of information sharing is important. Find the time to do Learner Exercise 9.7 to find out more about this aspect of your practice in your work setting.

To conclude

Earlier we encouraged you to complete Learner Exercise 9.2 and to identify aspects of your knowledge, skills and judgement related to information sharing. We also said that this was a *before and after* type of learning activity. Now is a good time to repeat the exercise and

Learner Exercise 9.7: Information sharing in your practice

Find out about information sharing in your area of practice.

In what areas of the overall activity are service users most likely to encounter failures to join up dots? Think about micro, meso and macro (individual, immediate team and wider organization) levels.

Are there simple interventions that can improve information sharing?

What are your own development needs with respect to information sharing?

Box 9.7: Further reading suggestions

Chapter 11, 'The Expression of Concerns by Individuals and Reaction to Those Concerns', and Chapter 12, 'Responses to Concerns and Actions Taken, and Whether Such Actions were Appropriate and Prompt', in Kennedy et al. (2001) *Learning from Bristol: The Report of the Public Inquiry into Children's Heart Surgery at the Bristol Royal Infirmary 1984–1995*, Command Paper CM 5207 also available at: <www.bristol-inquiry.org.uk/index.htm>.

This should help develop your appreciation of the difficulties noted in this chapter, in the section 'Many knew but it was too difficult to say'.

Remember also that there is a wide range of information and useful resources on the Every Child Matters: Change for Children website: <www.everychildmatters.co.uk>.

reflect on any differences in your responses. How has your thinking and understanding changed and developed? Do you know more now? Are you more aware of what you don't know – particularly in relation to your practice setting? If you want to find out more, then we suggest you read the material listed in Box 9.7.

We think that sharing information is one of the biggest challenges that you are likely to meet as an interprofessional practitioner. So we have summarized in Box 9.8 (opposite) some key principles of this crucial aspect of interprofessional practice.

Box 9.8: Some key principles of information sharing for interprofessional practitioners

- Share sufficient factual and contextual information for others to do their work effectively: not an overwhelming quantity and not too little to enable people to act, appreciate the significance of certain factors and make informed judgements
- Adhere to agreed templates or procedures for making information exchange fit for purpose or, where these are absent, structure your information to make the important parts readily discernible; use vocabulary and symbols that others will understand
- Pass things on soon enough for them to be acted upon before deterioration outruns the team's ability to respond in a way that avoids long-lasting damage and escalating service provision costs
- State clearly what you think (opinion/diagnosis) and what you want from others
- Relay the information the recipient needs to function in their role effectively, again using vocabulary or symbols that they will understand
- Make sure you share information with the correct people
- Make reasonable checks on the accuracy of information
- Review information periodically so that you spot emerging patterns and any errors or oversights
- Reflect on your approachability; ask yourself if you are responsive and receptive when other people request advice, resources, informal help and guidance.

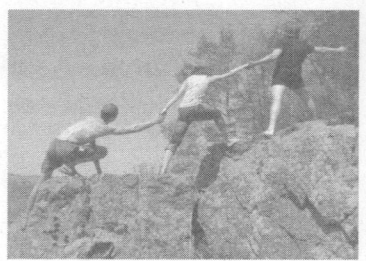

10

Being Interprofessional:
A Twenty-first-century
Career

My interest is in the future because I am going to spend the
rest of my life there.

Charles F. Kettering

What you will read in this chapter

This book was mostly written for learners on initial professional
education programmes, although we hope that qualified staff, carers
and users of services are also amongst our readers. Whoever you
are, we hope your career will progress and the ways in which you are
interprofessional develop. As these changes happen in the lives of
individuals, changes occur to organizations and ways of delivering
services: all with the aim that working interprofessionally will help to
deliver more effective public services. In this final chapter we put the
spotlight on two different aspects of change and development.

First, we focus on how being interprofessional changes as staff
develop and become more experienced at working and learning
about, from and with others. Recent graduates can contribute
a great deal to the workplace from their learning about being
interprofessional as a student. This needs nurturing as you become
part of the twenty-first-century (21C) workforce.

A job advert and a consultation call provide the basis for
an overview of different ways of working that you might meet.
Continuing professional development (CPD) plays an important part
in this. We suggest some CPD opportunities and how to participate in
the interprofessional community of practice.

Second, we briefly look beyond national boundaries to show some
of the many interprofessional initiatives already in place to enhance
services to international communities, and to provide optimal health
and social care in developing nations.

Being interprofessional: careers in the twenty-first century

Earlier we built a model to show what being interprofessional means. You may want to go back to the beginning to look at the models in chapter 1. Consider how your understanding of those models and being interprofessional has grown and become more sophisticated as you worked through different parts of this book. We are now interested in:

- How being interprofessional fits in with new and emerging roles, and ways of delivering public services; and
- What sort of service delivery teams a twenty-first-century interprofessional practitioner might be part of.

While thinking about these points, we spotted an advertisement in a university lift (Figure 10.1). Please take a few moments to study the advert and see how the birth centre is nested within a larger practice, alongside a range of other services. Then try to answer the following questions:

1 What range of practitioners will successful applicants for the advertised jobs be working with?
2 Why is this type of centre needed?
3 What is it replacing, and why?
4 What do they mean by multi-purpose rooms?
5 What will students need to learn that will help to make their curriculum vitae attractive to those who are recruiting staff for centres of this type?

With these questions in mind, we've designed Learner Exercises 10.1 and 10.2. The first is an interprofessional team-working exercise. The second is a personal task and can be done whether or not your particular area of practice relates to the advert. The focus is on the type of job, rather than the actual jobs in the Birth Centre, and on seeing yourself as being interprofessional and ready for new ways of working. We have assumed that you have either a Personal Development Plan (PDP) or Curriculum Vitae (CV), but don't worry if you haven't. Doing Learner Exercise 10.2 can be the start of either of these documents, or an entry in a portfolio of learning that you might use to demonstrate to others what you have learnt and what you can do.

Now we would like you to think about what you have learnt from this book and other interprofessional learning activities, and to gather evidence of this learning. In chapter 1 (Figure 1.1) we highlighted three key aspects of being interprofessional: thinking, feeling and doing (or acting). We said that being interprofessional meant knowing what to do, doing that in the correct way and having the appropriate attitudes, values and beliefs as we do it. We've built Learner Exercise 10.2 around this triangle of important elements of being interprofessional, as

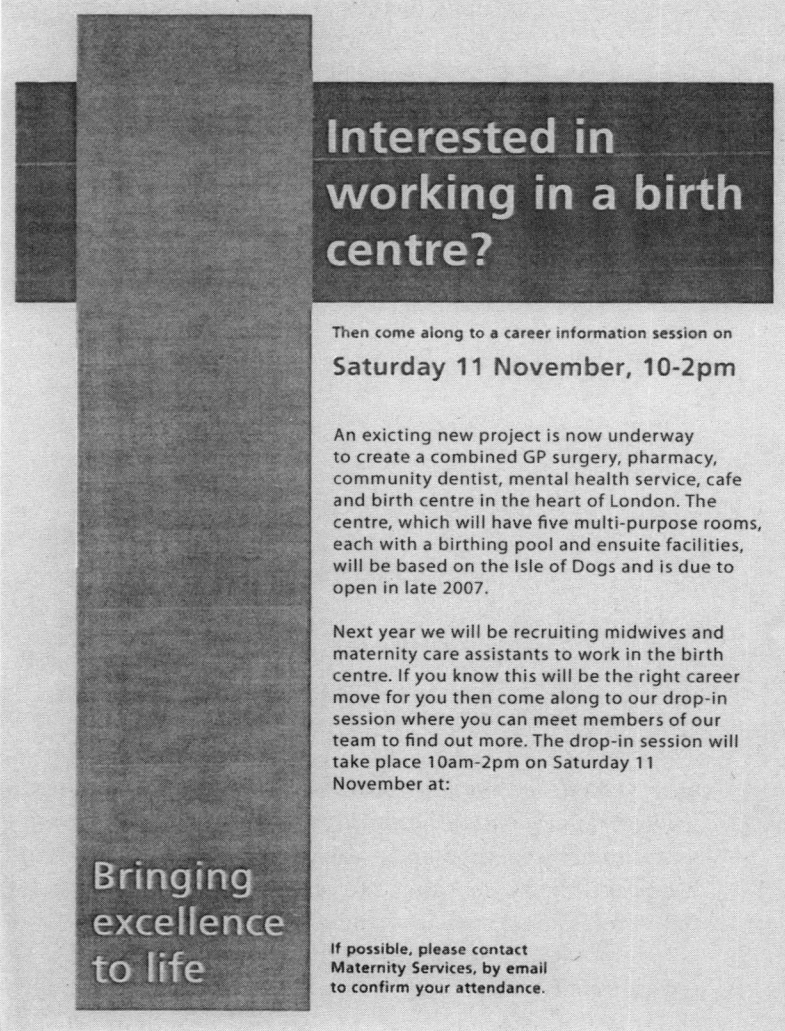

Interested in working in a birth centre?

Then come along to a career information session on

Saturday 11 November, 10-2pm

An exciting new project is now underway to create a combined GP surgery, pharmacy, community dentist, mental health service, cafe and birth centre in the heart of London. The centre, which will have five multi-purpose rooms, each with a birthing pool and ensuite facilities, will be based on the Isle of Dogs and is due to open in late 2007.

Next year we will be recruiting midwives and maternity care assistants to work in the birth centre. If you know this will be the right career move for you then come along to our drop-in session where you can meet members of our team to find out more. The drop-in session will take place 10am-2pm on Saturday 11 November at:

Bringing excellence to life

If possible, please contact Maternity Services, by email to confirm your attendance.

Figure 10.1 An interprofessional career opportunity

Learner Exercise 10.1: Mapping a team for a new way of working

Write a list of everyone who might learn and work in the Birth Centre.

Look at the advert side by side with your list: are there additional things that could be said to make the advert more reflective of who is in your list?

Discuss why the advert says that the Birth Centre is 'an exciting new project'.

List the people who will be using the Birth Centre; now reflect on whether there are staff missing from your first list whose services these people might need? Some of the things we wrote about in chapter 8 are worth considering here.

Discuss some things that could help ensure that staff in the Birth Centre work collaboratively and feel satisfied with their jobs.

we think that it's valuable to give evidence of your capabilities for all three aspects. We've put in one example for each to show what we mean. You may like to store your answers to Exercise 10.2 in a place where they will be easy to find the next time you apply for a job or find yourself preparing for a selection interview. It may be a while before you need to synthesize and present evidence of your capabilities in collaborative working, and re-reading the book and your notes may be a helpful reminder of things you have learnt and practised.

Learner Exercise 10.2: Putting together a being-interprofessional curriculum vitae

My Interprofessional curriculum vitae

1. **What I know about being interprofessional.** Remember that knowing the advantages of working in this way and knowing what problems can arise because of its complexity are equally important.
   For example:
   It means working with someone who has a different practice or works differently to me . . .
   . . . .
   . . . .
   . . . .

2. **What I have done that involved being interprofessional and working collaboratively with others.** This could be as part of your studies in an interprofessional module or when you were on a work attachment or placement. Be as specific as you can: state what the task was, what role you had, what interprofessional skills you applied, etc.
   For example:
   In our learning group I reminded everyone that different perspectives don't have to be in competition with one another but can be complementary or constructively challenging . . .
   . . . .
   . . . .
   . . . .

3. **I approach working with others interprofessionally by . . .**
   For example:
   Showing respect for the pace of others' work, as the pace of my work seems to be different . . .
   . . . .
   . . . .
   . . . .

Instead of presenting this as a list, you can also join up the three aspects and write an account of a particular interprofessional experience that includes what was done, why it was done that way and how it was done. It doesn't have to be very long; just make sure you show what you know, and did and felt, about being interprofessional.

Box 10.1: A setting for interprofessional working

Strategic Plan for Reducing Re-offending 2008–11

The Ministry of Justice is inviting comments on the government's new and overarching three-year strategic plan to reduce re-offending. The draft plan sets out a number of key questions for respondents to consider. These include:

How do we ensure continuity of care between adult and youth justice services?
How do we ensure today's young offenders don't become adult offenders?
How can local agencies work more effectively together to reduce re-offending?

The consultation also asks whether there is particular scope for more joined-up work around parenting and family-oriented interventions delivered by Youth Offending Teams and in response to domestic violence.

(<http://noms.justice.gov.uk/news-publications-events/publications/consultations>;
accessed 21 January 2008)

Now we turn to a different setting for interprofessional working. Our choice is deliberate: to show that this way of working applies in many different settings. We think most of your experience to date will have been face to face with others. Sometimes that is not possible or practical, or not even necessary. Arranging for different practitioners to contribute their knowledge and views on a subject is another way of harnessing the strength of the interprofessional team.

In the example we use in Box 10.1 – a call for comment on proposals for new ways of reducing re-offending in the UK – the idea was to gather multiple views virtually. The government was proposing a strategy or plan and inviting anyone to offer suggestions about how to ensure it will work in practice. Notice that they have already identified the need for more 'joined-up work' and suggested the need for some continuity between adult and youth justice services. Readers of this book will hardly be surprised by this. We've shown in the previous chapters that interprofessional working for staff and agencies offers a practical way of providing more effective services for almost all service users. Others have written in more detail about collaborative working in a youth crime team (Anning et al. 2006).

Take a moment to read the three questions in Box 10.1 in the context of your learning about what it means to be interprofessional, to work collaboratively with colleagues from different work settings, and for agencies to join up their services. We think you will know a great deal that could help the people whose job it will be to put this plan of the government into action. Make some notes about what you would offer as comments, possibly using headings such as:

- Practitioners needed for this type of work with young people
- The agencies they presently work for

- *Ways to support* staff working in the redesigned services.
- . . .

Of course, this virtual way of working has its downsides: remember our comments about levels of participation in chapter 8. What do you think are the downsides of virtual consultation? What are the best ways of making sure that all the relevant members of the interprofessional team contribute?

Working in the ways we've outlined above means paying attention to our personal and professional development, so that as we have increasing responsibility and participate in different models of collaborative working we maintain and develop our capability to be interprofessional. Many documents set out competencies and capability in the different areas of practice and for all the professions. As an example we've selected the development of Ten Essential Shared Capabilities by an interprofessional national steering group who established a framework for all mental health practitioners that spans their career. You can see this in Box 10.2 (p. 194). Even if your practice brings you into contact with different service users, the headings used in this framework will still be relevant to you. They may seem to be common sense and at the

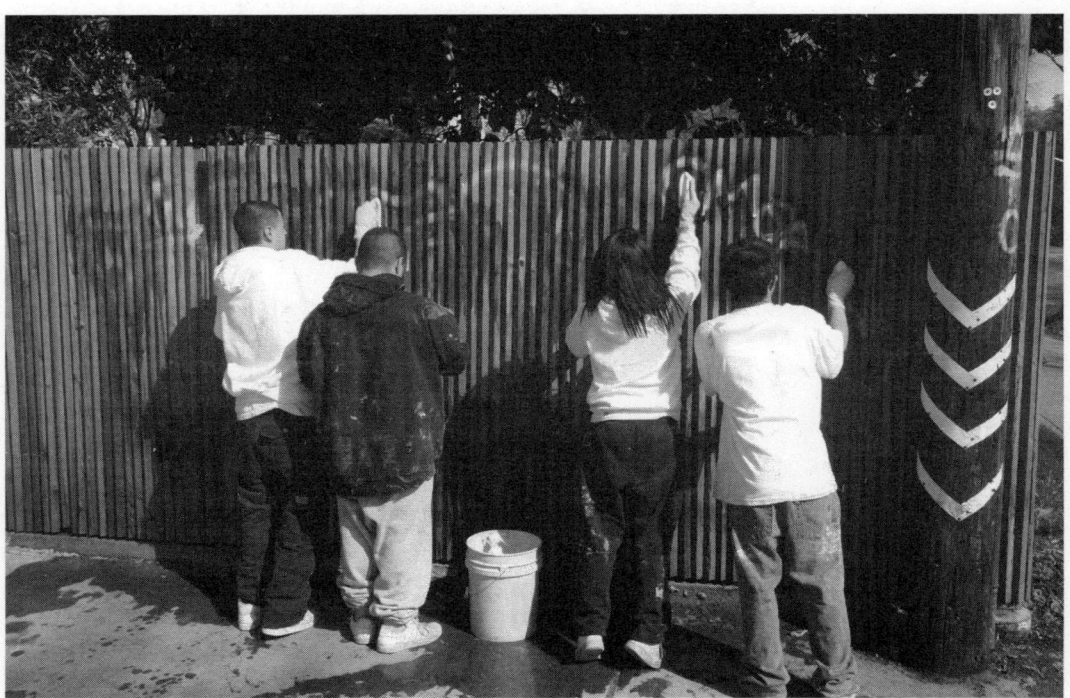

Photo 10.1 A community-service initiative aimed at young offenders; can you think of examples from your area of practice that could help the Ministry of Justice's goals to reduce re-offending among young people? Rick Rhay/iStock.

same time aspirational. You might think as you read the list of bolded headings:

I already do this, it's just part of my usual practice.

You might also think:

Goodness, this is a list of tough things to get right all the time.

We suggest you put these first reactions aside and find time to consider the suggestions we make in Learner Exercise 10.3. You can do this by yourself but, as we've suggested in other places, this book is about being interprofessional so if you can, make this a piece of team work. The work in Learner Exercise 10.3 is not easy, and sharing your reflections with people you learn and work with can be difficult. You might not want them to know some of your answers. An alternative way of approaching this exercise is to use the ten points to assess how an interprofessional team works. Ask what the team's strengths are, and where more needs to be done by the team for capable and effective practice. If you are learning and working collaboratively with a long-standing team you might like to suggest that the team undertakes Interprofessional Development Planning (IPDP).

You may already have a PDP, and be familiar with the development process that these encourage in relation to other aspects of your learning and practice as a student and employee. Many institutions and organizations require you to have a PDP that shows how you identify the ways you wish to develop, the development work you have done and what this has achieved. For those of you unfamiliar with PDPs, Pause Point 10.1 has some key features of these. For information about PDPs for your work, you can get in touch with your professional or registration body and the human resources department in your organization.

Learner Exercise 10.3: Being interprofessional: assessing capability

Make a note of the essential skills and capabilities in Box 10.1 that relate to being interprofessional.

Reflect on your strengths and 'not so' strengths for each one. You could use a five-star system for this.

Link this work with your Personal Development Plan by identifying:

- What skills need most attention
- How much time you have to develop these skills
- The ways in which you can improve these skills.

Remember to return to your assessment to look at what other skills you also need to develop.

Pause Point 10.1: The PDP

The PDP (in brief) is:

- Yours: to be shared only with others of your choice
- A way of taking responsibility for your development
- A record of your personal development planning process
- Either written or kept electronically
- Evidence of your development and your skills that can be used as part of a job application.

We are suggesting that the IPDP is a way for interprofessional teams to identify a team's development needs and how to meet these. The quote below is an excerpt from the Quality Assurance Agency for England's Statement of Common Purpose, about values in relation to cooperation and collaboration with colleagues, for health and social care practitioners. You could use these to start a discussion about what the focus of an IPDP for your team should be.

Health and social care staff should:

- respect and encourage the skills and contributions which colleagues in both their own profession and other professions bring to the care of clients and patients
- within their work environment, support colleagues to develop their professional knowledge, skills and performance
- not require colleagues to take on responsibilities that are beyond their level of knowledge, skills and experience.

(*Statement of Common Purpose for Subject Benchmark Statements for the Health and Social Care Professions*, Quality Assurance Agency for Higher Education for England (undated))

It often helps if a team can get away from its usual workplace to work on its development. A team 'away day', perhaps facilitated by someone from outside the team and involving participation in workshops, allows everyone to focus on interprofessional capabilities. There are facilitators and organizations that offer this, but if you want to organize interprofessional learning for your own team then there is a range of useful resources, including Freeth et al. (2005), Freeth (2007), and Hammick et al. (2009).

The essential capabilities in Box 10.2 are applicable across a range of practitioners and, as we noted above, not only for those working with mental health service users. We now want to extend these and say a little more about some of the key features of being interprofessional that we discussed in earlier chapters. Our sights are on the interprofessional competences of a mid-career practitioner

Box 10.2: The Ten Essential Shared Capabilities for Mental Health Practice

Working in Partnership. Developing and maintaining constructive working relationships with service users, carers, families, colleagues, lay people and wider community networks. Working positively with any tensions created by conflicts of interest or aspiration that may arise between the partners in care.

Respecting Diversity. Working in partnership with service users, carers, families and colleagues to provide care and interventions that not only make a positive difference but also do so in ways that respect and value diversity including age, race, culture, disability, gender, spirituality and sexuality.

Practising Ethically. Recognising the rights and aspirations of service users and their families, acknowledging power differentials and minimising them whenever possible. Providing treatment and care that is accountable to service users and carers within the boundaries prescribed by national (professional), legal and local codes of ethical practice.

Challenging Inequality. Addressing the causes and consequences of stigma, discrimination, social inequality and exclusion on service users, carers and mental health services. Creating, developing or maintaining valued social roles for people in the communities they come from.

Promoting Recovery. Working in partnership to provide care and treatment that enables service users and carers to tackle mental health problems with hope and optimism and to work towards a valued lifestyle within and beyond the limits of any mental health problem.

Identifying People's Needs and Strengths. Working in partnership to gather information to agree health and social care needs in the context of the preferred lifestyle and aspirations of service users, their families, carers and friends.

Providing Service User Centred Care. Negotiating achievable and meaningful goals; primarily from the perspective of service users and their families. Influencing and seeking the means to achieve these goals and clarifying the responsibilities of the people who will provide any help that is needed, including systematically evaluating outcomes and achievements.

Making a Difference. Facilitating access to and delivering the best quality, evidence-based, values-based health and social care interventions to meet the needs and aspirations of service users and their families and carers.

Promoting Safety and Positive Risk Taking. Empowering the person to decide the level of risk they are prepared to take with their health and safety. This includes working with the tension between promoting safety and positive risk taking, including assessing and dealing with possible risks for service users, carers, family members, and the wider public.

Personal Development and Learning. Keeping up-to-date with changes in practice and participating in life-long learning, personal and professional development for one's self and colleagues through supervision, appraisal and reflective practice.

(Hope 2004, p. 3)

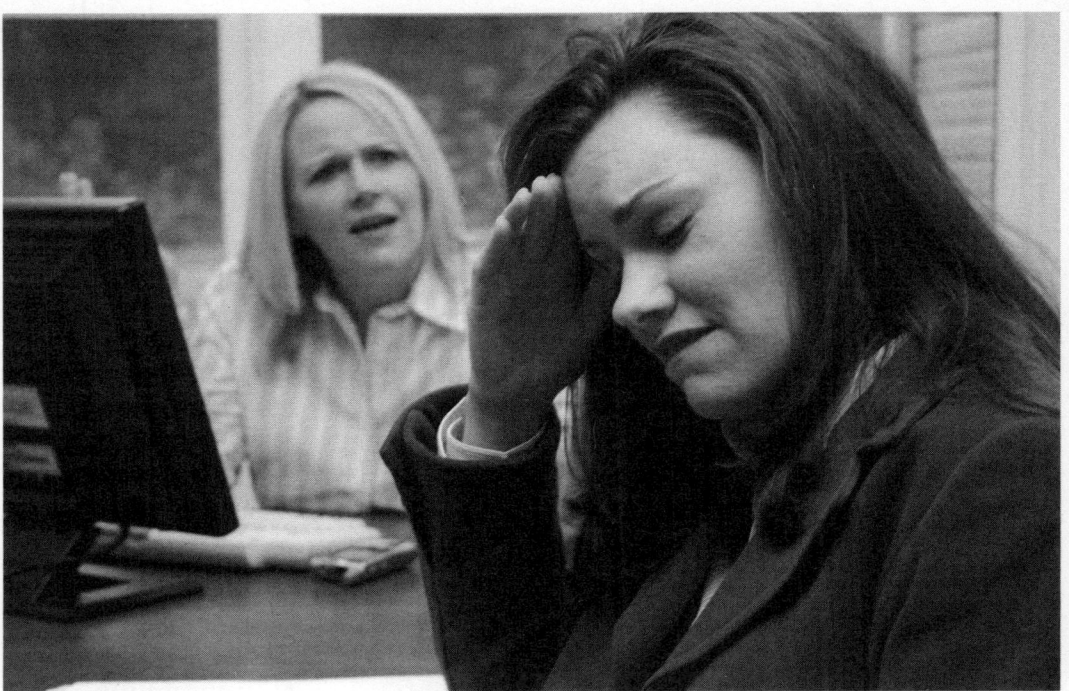

Photo 10.2 Conflict can arise in a team; what do you feel are the central skills needed to avoid and resolve conflict? Brad Killer/iStock.

rather than first-post interprofessional competences for newly qualified staff. Our concern is with what more senior members of the interprofessional team might be expected to be capable of and in this way show new team members the ways collaborative working is effective. We would again emphasize that this way of working has its challenges. The quote below relates being interprofessional to being an artist in a troop or group, and reminds us that relating to others in these complex ways demands more than just the ordinary aspects of work relationships. For example, as remarked by Soubhi (2007, p. 14), it calls for harmony. So what helps the harmony of an interprofessional working team?

> . . . professionals pursue universal human goals: to survive and fulfil their potential. They create their own ways of connecting formally and informally with colleagues, patients, and families; they define – implicitly or explicitly – their own goals depending on the situation at hand. Above all, they undergo, not only through formal conferences and teachings, but also through informal interactions with colleagues and circumstances, a learning process akin to what happens in a theatre troop or a jazz ensemble where each player harmonises their play according to what the others are playing.

In the same way that jazz playing requires more than just instruments and musical skills, IPE requires more than just curricula and teaching resources. IPE is about living communities of professionals; it is about mutual dependencies among the participants in care delivery – professionals, patients and family members – and it is about how these participants can successfully face daily challenges to adjust care strategies according to the demands of patients' illnesses and the resources to meet them. (Soubhi, 2007, *Newsletter of The Network: Towards Unity For Health* 26 (2 December 2007)

Our assertions about interprofessional learning and working, and the examples we chose to illustrate these, show that contributions to interprofessional harmony come from people who have knowledge of, are skilful in, and have the appropriate attitudes to:

- Leadership
- Followership
- Interdependent decision-making
- Reflective practice
- Conflict management
- Confidence to question yourself and others
- Collective responsibility.

We have already touched on some of the attributes in the above list because sometimes even newly qualified staff have, for example, to lead an interprofessional team, as the scenarios in chapter 5 show. Others need cultivating as you become more experienced and take more responsibility for the harmony of the interprofessional team.

We now look at conflict resolution, having the confidence to question yourself and others, and collective responsibility. To do this, we take up the story that started in chapter 5 by revisiting the final two scenes.

In scene 4 our novice practitioner was impressed by the way the chair of the case conference managed the situation when the results of a client's assessment were not ready. You might like to read this section of chapter 5 again now if you've forgotten the details. When this fact was discovered, the chair ensured both that the people present did not start to attribute blame for this *and* that the error was not repeated. In other words, she prevented any conflict arising at the meeting – probably the best way to manage conflict is not to let it happen in the first place! Second, she made sure a similar situation did not occur again for that client by asking someone to take responsibility for obtaining the results. Another positive way to prevent conflict in a team is to make sure everyone is clear about what their responsibilities are. Third, the chair then organized a working group to address any failures in the system for ensuring results were ready in time for case conferences. She is seeking a resolution by bringing people together so that they can learn about the problem and work together to solve it. You might recognize this as being very like problem-based learning – an approach that works well for an interprofessional team. As we said before, the *problem* is a gap in what we know: working together to identify what we need to know is the first step towards learning about the solution.

When the working group meets, its members will have to learn about each other (remember that all groups or teams start with the Forming or getting to know each other stage – see chapter 4). Then it's likely that they will need to learn from each other about the reasons why assessment results may not be available at a case conference. Let's hope that the working group is chaired by someone as skilled as the case conference chair; someone who makes sure that everyone has their turn to speak and listens to what their colleagues say. Finding out why things happen and exactly what people want helps to find a resolution that suits everyone.

Conflicts are mostly solved by meeting individual (and in this case it might be an individual agency) and collective needs. It is also important to be user-focused in this situation: after all, their needs are the most important ones. All these needs have to be explicit if they are to be met. This may mean that the working-group members have to ask questions about their own practice and about others' practice. For example, the person responsible for organizing the case conference might need to ask if s/he takes the capacity of the regional assessment centre into account when the date is organized. Does the assessment centre know the importance of the case conference for the service user? Staff at the regional assessment centre might need to ask themselves if they really see the results in terms of a client, or if the end result is just a set of facts. Do their colleagues know how they work and how much time the assessments take? The capability of everyone involved to ask these types of questions, and actively use the answers to find a solution will lead to a successful outcome of the working group.

Finally, the hard work of the group will only be successful if the solution is put into routine practice. This is likely to require everyone involved to change their own practice in some way and for everyone involved to work together. This means taking collective responsibility for a new way of doing things and possibly asking other colleagues to work in this way too. It is often hard to keep to agreements made in a working group like this when you return to your place of work. It becomes your turn to manage the hostility that introducing change can evoke. Maintaining contact with working-group colleagues through an action-learning set can help to support you as you endeavour to convince people of the need for change in your separate workplaces.

Action learning is 'a continuous process of learning and reflection that happens with the support of. . .colleagues, working on real issues with the intention of getting things done' (McGill and Brockbank 2004, p. 11). Action-learning sets are similar, then, to interprofessional teams using real-life problems for effective learning about, from and with each other, and creating the conditions for collaboration.

In this section we've highlighted some of the ways conflicts can be prevented and resolved. Resolution often depends on meeting the challenge of being able to ask yourself and others difficult questions. This way of learning and working involves taking collective responsibility, and we looked at ways to find support as you do this. Other ways of finding support and maintaining your interprofessional competencies are outlined next.

One professional aspect of being interprofessional is keeping up-to-date with developments in interprofessional learning and working. It's useful to see this as an integral part of your CPD alongside all the other profession-specific topics you need to keep abreast of. We've put a few suggestions about sources of knowledge on interprofessional matters in Box 10.3.

Having extended the view to look at different ways of working interprofessionally, and how your interprofessional practice might develop to more advanced stages of working in this way, we now turn briefly to what interprofessional collaboration looks like internationally.

Box 10.3: Finding out more about being interprofessional

Ways to find out about evidence-based interprofessional practice

The Social Care Institute for Excellence <www.scie.org.uk>
The Cochrane Collaboration <www.cochrane.org>
The Campbell Collaboration <www.campbellcollaboration.org>

Journals that have articles about being interprofessional

International Journal of Integrated Care <http://www.ijic.org>
Journal of Integrated Care <http://www.pavpub.com/pavpub/journals/JIC/index.asp>
Journal of Interprofessional Care <www.tandf.co.uk/journals/titles>

Conferences that focus on interprofessional education and collaborative working

All Together Better Health – a bi-annual international conference.

Organizations with an interest in being interprofessional

CAIPE United Kingdom Interprofessional Students Network <www.caipe.org.uk>
The International Network of Integrated Care <http://www.integratedcarenetwork.org>
The Network Towards Unity for Health <www.the-networktufh.org>

Being interprofessional: a global view

In most of this book we have used examples from the UK: a decision linked to where we think most of our readers are learning and working. Three aspects of this need attention. First, this is not to ignore the global interprofessional community of practice. In previous chapters, amongst the more local examples you will have found some mention of the international nature of learning and working interprofessionally.

Second, our readers may be presently in the UK. This does not mean that is where they were born and raised, and neither does it mean that is where they will live for the rest of their working lives. As you read this final chapter, you may be planning a career move to another European Union country; or farther afield to one of the many countries where the capability to be interprofessional is an essential for those delivering public services such as social care, education and public health.

Third, in the spirit of learning interprofessionally, there is much to learn about the way public services are delivered in other countries. This happens at governmental levels with official overseas visits from ministers (usually those who are newly appointed) searching for different (and often more economic) ways of achieving effectiveness. Practitioner and academic exchanges take place so that people can see and discuss developments. In a wide range of contexts, people write or present what they learnt about and from others. You can probably list other ways to learn from other countries (Voluntary Service Overseas, Special Study Modules on placement abroad) and, of course, if you can't actually travel, then a <www> search is a good alternative.

Boxes 10.4, 10.5 and 10.6 showcase some activities in different parts of the world that embrace the concept of being interprofessional. The example from Newfoundland shows how interprofessional learning and working are possible and valuable for practitioners serving a remote rural community through video-conferencing (Box 10.4). This is a way of creating a community of interprofessional practice when face-to-face meetings are impractical. Note the diverse practitioners mentioned in the developments showcased in Box 10.5, and how the examples are based in the community. We think that these examples have a message about always asking who should be in the interprofessional team. Our last international example (Box 10.6) was chosen because it reflects much of what we wrote about in Part II of the book. It shows the importance of asking about what works and what doesn't work in complex partnership arrangements, and how evaluation is used to make changes that result in improvements. We hope our selection gives you the appetite to do more international learning about, from and with others.

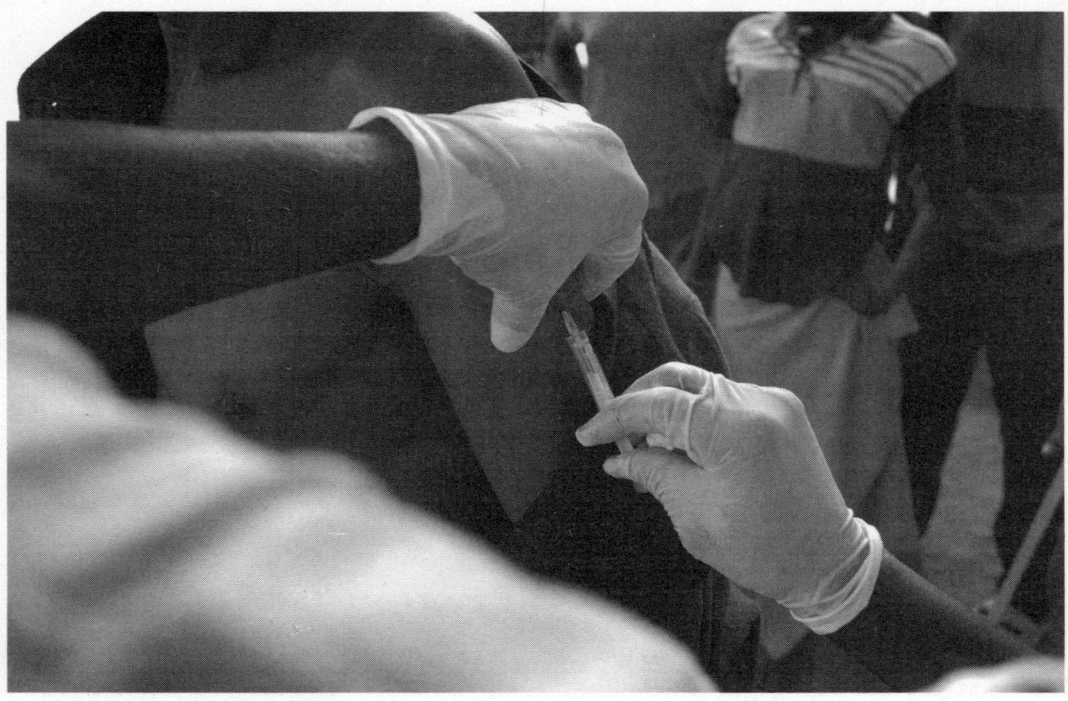

Photo 10.3 Although many aspects of collaborative work are transferable to worldwide contexts, working overseas offers great opportunities for learning new lessons about interprofessional work which can enrich your practice. Sean Warren/iStock.

Box 10.4: Rural Mental Health Interprofessional Training Programme at Memorial University, Newfoundland and Labrador, Canada

A programme was developed to focus on interprofessional, collaborative practice skills in six critical domains of mental health practice.

Participants in both communities came from several professions: social work, nursing, police, family medicine, community mental health, emergency medicine, long term care, school counselors, and clergy. They reported the need to increase their knowledge of mental health issues and inadequate referral sources in the community as the main reasons for attending the training. They emphasized the socio-economic problems facing rural communities, the need for assistance when working with alcohol, drug, and gambling addictions, and inadequate educational opportunities for health professionals.

Analysis of the evaluation data indicated a positive response and the value of interprofessional collaboration. Participants reported a high level of confidence in their ability to work collaboratively with other professions, to deal with situations of conflict, and develop interdisciplinary care plans for patients. Specifically, according to pre and post testing, participants increased their belief that patients receiving team care are more likely to be treated as whole persons.

Of the eighteen mental health issues addressed, eating disorders, addictions, sexual assault, and child sexual abuse saw the largest increases in participant confidence.

Once participants became familiar with video-conferencing they found a level of comfort communicating through this media. Despite some challenges in the delivery of the video-conferencing, there was an overall appreciation of this type of training that would otherwise be very difficult to provide to rural areas.

(<http://www.mun.ca/rmhitp/synopsis.php>; accessed 10 September 2008)

Box 10.5: Global examples of interprofessional education and team-working

Interprofessional education has been reported in a wide range of developing countries, including Algeria, the Cameroons, the Dominican Republic, Fiji, the Philippines, Thailand, the Sudan, Beirut, Columbia and South Africa. Some of these initiatives are similar to those reported in developed countries. Others extend the range of professions to include, for example, agriculturists, engineers and sanitarians engaged in public health and community development projects. Some are also designed to create a flexible workforce that the country can afford, unfettered by narrow definitions of professionalism and preconceived demarcations inherited from colonial powers.

(Adapted from: Meads and Barr 2005, p. 143)

Collaborative practice in Brazil

In 1993 the Brazilian government introduced the health-care networks within which family health teams work in primary care units. These teams are composed of a doctor, one nurse, one or two nursing assistants, and five to six community health agents, and are responsible for a maximum of 4,000 people. Their work includes health promotion, prevention, restoration and rehabilitation of frequent diseases and disorders. The design has led to a significant improvement in health care and in the quality of life of the Brazilian people.

(Adapted from:
<http://dtr2004.saude.gov.br/dab/docs/eventos/3a_mostra/nota_tecnica_mostra_ingles.pdf>; accessed 29 August 2008)

Interprofessional learning and team work in diabetes care, Hibbing, United States

Because of the sizeable geriatric population of the community, the low-income levels of the population, high rates of obesity, and the increase in the incidence of Type 2 diabetes, Fairview Mesaba Clinics (FMC) /Range Regional Health Services (RRHS) identified diabetes as their community-based initiative. The Diabetes Education interprofessional team consists of three nurses (two of whom are Certified Diabetes Educators or CDE), two dietitians (one is CDE), a pharmacist, and a primary care provider. Students in RPAP medicine, dentistry, pharmacy and nursing are involved in the project. Students help develop portions of the diabetes education classes and assist with health screening. The project later expanded to work more closely with the clinics responsible for diagnosing and educating patients about cardiovascular disease.

Working and learning together in North Minneapolis, United States

The Broadway Clinic in North Minneapolis received funding in 2008 to address the complex set of issues presented by the clinic's patients. The community of North Minneapolis is a medically under-served, lower socio-economic community whose members have fewer resources than average. There is a high prevalence of unemployment in the community. Most patients presenting to the clinic have multiple medical problems, all impacted by their economic status and community resources. The Broadway Clinic team consists of family physicians, a psychiatrist, a pharmacist, a nurse practitioner, a social worker, a dental student, a marriage and family therapist, and a psychologist. All the above are on staff and have extensive training in their field, and at least three years of education experience. Students from all of the above professions are welcome and will work together with staff, assisting with problem identification and to implement solutions.

(Both case studies from the United States were adapted from: <http://www.mnahec.umn.edu/AHEC/about/Interprofessional_Education_Sites.html>; accessed 29 August 2008)

Box 10.6: Rural health in the United States – enhancing community university partnerships in a rural state

We are a team of psychiatrists, family physicians, social workers and trainees from the University of New Mexico (UNM) who travel throughout the state of New Mexico, responding to requests for consultations from community residents and care providers to see individuals who have intellectual disabilities with complex medical, behavioural, and psychiatric problems. We treat these individuals in their own communities: at their homes, doctor's offices, agencies, job sites, and day programmes. In the process, we provide training to learners from the university as well as community caregivers, physicians, and agency providers. Fundamentally, we model respectful interviewing and physical exams with patients who are often non-verbal and sometimes fairly agitated. Family members and extensive support teams are welcome to participate; they provide essential information and are often role models for us. The programme is funded by the State of New Mexico and is based at the University of New Mexico Health Sciences Centre. We have 14 years of experience doing this work and over the years have been able to sort out what works and what does not work in our quest to develop sustainable partnerships between the university and the communities we visit.

Some strategies that consistently work:

- Respond to a need that the community requests rather than offer something that the university wants. Community members consistently complain that university visitors are far too often searching for research subjects than answering needs.
- Designate a university-based contact person who is accessible to community members, and who is committed to returning phone calls and emails.
- Find out what is already successful and build on it, rather than giving presumed 'expert advice'. Be sure that you function as a consultant, rather than a judgmental visitor.
- Offer and help facilitate access to special resources that the university may offer.

Using Telecommunications

It is always important to establish a face-to face, community-to-community relationship first, and then use telecommunication as a way to continue the conversation, consultation, or patient evaluation. It is easy to assume that the technology will solve all rural access problems, but often poor understanding of equipment capacity, technological failures, and lack of communication between sites lead to dashed hopes. Realistic expectations should be made clear from the beginning so problems that arise do not become overwhelming. The university should provide technical assistance and try to solve technical glitches so that solutions do not cost the community extra money.

Effective Training Across Disciplines

Unlike traditional post-graduate education, that is very lecture-based and discipline specific, our faculty consciously model a team approach that trains students to function well in an interprofessional process. Long car rides to rural areas and shared meals shape the team and cement bonds within the team. We had several unsuccessful attempts to link with community health providers. Failed early educational attempts included newsletters to practicing clinicians that went unread and assigned student visits to patients' homes without adequate faculty support. As students and residents graduate from UNM and establish their own practices, they feel comfortable caring for individuals with intellectual disabilities, and often serve as the local resource to other providers.

Patient Success Enhances Partnerships

Seeing patients in their own homes and work sites removes the added stress of having to drive for several hours to see the team at the university. Patients and families are welcoming and proud to show us their homes, hobbies, and successes. Care givers are happier and are able to enhance their abilities to care for their own patients.

Getting Results

Graduates of this community-focused training process tell us that their comfort level, confidence and competence in working with adults with intellectual disabilities in their home communities have soared. Many learners report that they are now willing to treat these clients in their communities and share their experience and expertise with colleagues; in the past, they would often avoid treating these patients. Clients do not need institutional care, prolonged hospitalization, or frequent trips to the University Hospital to get the same excellent care. These university-community partnerships in training and service have served as fertile ground to improve healthcare throughout the state for individuals with intellectual disabilities and complex medical, psychiatric and behavioural problems.

(Silverblatt and Seeger 2007, p. 11)

To conclude

Our central focus in this chapter has been the interprofessional practitioner moving into their workplace as a member of staff rather than as a student. In harmony with the jazz metaphor used by Soubhi (2007), we have extended and elaborated many aspects of being interprofessional that we touched on in previous chapters. Our emphasis has been on the importance, for the soloist and the team, of continuous learning and nurturing so that the harmony of being interprofessional is maintained. In this way learning about, from and with each other, and working collaboratively, become an effective means of improving the well-being of all service users.

Glossary

anti-discriminatory practice
Ensures that people's ability to achieve their potential is not limited by prejudice or discrimination. There is respect for and protection of each individual's human rights and respect for the dignity and worth of each individual. Each individual has an equal opportunity to participate in society, and there is mutual respect between groups based on understanding and valuing of diversity and on shared respect for equality and human rights (<http://www.cehr.org.uk/content/objectives.rhtm>).

ASSIA
Applied Social Sciences Index and Abstracts, an indexing and abstracting tool covering the literature in health, social services, psychology, sociology, economics, politics, race relations and education.

CINHAL
The Combined Index of Nursing and Allied Health Literature database.

collaboration
An active and ongoing partnership, often between people from diverse backgrounds, who work together to solve problems or provide services and share experiences. It differs from cooperation and coordination, which are less elaborate and ambitious ways of working together. Being cooperative means being open, willing and available to work with others, and when undertaking coordination activities people focus primarily on the timing and sequencing of working together.

collaborative practice
When multiple workers from different professional backgrounds provide comprehensive services by working together synergistically, along with service users, their families, carers and communities, to deliver care.

continuing professional development (CPD)	A planned and organized approach to your learning after initial qualification. Practitioners from many work settings are required by statutory and professional bodies to do a certain amount of CPD each year to maintain the registration that permits them to practice.
Curriculum Vitae	The organized and concise presentation of details about yourself to show your education, work experience and capabilities in a clear timeline. It is often presented in addition to an application job form. Résumé is another term used for something that is very similar.
enquiry-based learning (EBL)	An alternative term for problem-based learning, sometimes preferred to avoid negative connotations of the word 'problem'.
equal opportunity	A descriptive term for an approach to provide an environment in which people are not excluded from the activities of society, such as education and health and social care, on the basis of immutable traits (adapted from <http://en.wikipedia.org/wiki/Equal_ opportunities>).
ERIC	A US-based Education Resources Information Centre that gives free access to more than 1.2 million bibliographic records of journal articles and other education-related materials and, if available, includes links to full text.
expert patient programmes	Aim to help patients with long-term and/ or chronic conditions gain life skills and, with proper support, to take the lead in 'self-managing' their conditions. For more information, see <http://www.expertpatients. nhs.uk/>.
Green Paper	In Britain, the Republic of Ireland and other similar Commonwealth jurisdictions (e.g., Australia), a Green Paper is a tentative government report of a proposal, without any commitment to action; the first step in changing the law. Green Papers may result in the production of a White Paper. See <http://en.wikipedia.org/wiki/Green_paper>, for a description of a European Union Green Paper, and below for a description of a White Paper.

ideology A set of beliefs, ideas or doctrines that reflects the thinking of a given cultural, social, political or economic group, or of an individual.

Medline A literature-indexing service in medicine and related fields, provided by the US National Library of Medicine.

patient pathway The route that a patient will take from their first contact with a member of staff in health services, through referral, to the completion of their treatment. It can be seen as a timeline, on which every event relating to treatment such as consultations, diagnosis, treatment, medication, diet, assessment, teaching and preparing for discharge from the hospital can all be mapped
(adapted from <http://www.dh.gov.uk/en/ Policyandguidance/Organisationpolicy/ Secondarycare/Treatmentcentres/index.htm>).

patient-centred care Explores the patient's main reason for the visit, concerns, and need for information; seeks an integrated understanding of the patient's world – that is, their whole person, emotional needs and life issues, and finds common ground on what the problem is and mutually agrees on management. It aims to enhance prevention and health promotion, and the continuing relationship between the patient and the doctor (adapted from Stewart 2001, Towards a Global Definition of Patient Centred Care, *British Medical Journal* 322: 444–5).

personal development plan (PDP) A collection of documents which record your progress in meeting your identified learning and development needs, and shows the activities you have undertaken to meet these needs and your achievements.

problem-based learning (PBL) A way of delivering a curriculum in order to develop problem-solving skills, as well as assisting learners with the acquisition of necessary skills. Learners work cooperatively in groups to seek solutions to real-world problems, set to engage their curiosity and initiate learning the subject matter.

strategy High-level planning for a service or organizations, involving goal-setting and budgeting.

White Papers	Issued by the government and set out policy, or proposed action, on a topic of current concern. Although a White Paper may on occasion be a consultation as to the details of new legislation, it does signify a clear intention on the part of a government to pass new laws. See <http://en.wikipedia.org/wiki/White_paper> for more details.
World Health Organisation (WHO)	The directing and coordinating authority for health within the United Nations system. It is responsible for providing leadership on global health matters, shaping the health research agenda, setting norms and standards, articulating evidence-based policy options, providing technical support to countries, and monitoring and assessing health trends. For more details, see <http://www.who.int>.

Appendix: Some Interprofessional Organizations

AIPPEN The Australasian Interprofessional Practice and Education Network, founded at the All Together Better Health 3 Conference in London in 2006.

CAIPE The Centre for the Advancement of Interprofessional Education is a charity and company, limited by guarantee, whose claim to special expertise is founded on its members, publications and development activities. Its members form a network of mutual support and interest that facilitates intellectual engagement with, and the development of, individual and organizational interprofessionalism. CAIPE promotes and develops interprofessional education as a way of improving collaboration between practitioners and organizations, engaged in both statutory and non-statutory public services and improving the quality of care that is delivered to the public. It supports the integration of health and social care in local communities. CAIPE is a UK and international authoritative voice on interprofessional education in universities and the workplace across health and social care; <http://www.caipe.org.uk>.

CCPH Community-Campus Partnerships for Health is a US not-for-profit organization that promotes health through partnerships between communities and higher educational institutions; <http://www.ccph.info/>.

CEIMH Centre of Excellence in Interdisciplinary Mental Health. Based at the University of Birmingham, UK, this is a partnership between six university disciplines, key local, national and international mental health agencies, and service user and carer organizations; <http://www.ceimh.bham.ac.uk/> (accessed 9 September 2008).

CIHC The Canadian Interprofessional Health Collaborative is an initiative funded by Health Canada. It aims to promote and demonstrate the benefits of interprofessional education for collaborative patient-centred practice and to stimulate networking and the sharing of the best approaches to interprofessional education for collaborative patient-centred practice; <http://www.cihc.ca>.

DIPEx is a resource for patients, carers, family and friends, doctors, nurses and other health practitioners, set up in 2001 by two doctors after their own experience of illness. The website contains interviews with everyday people talking about their own experiences of serious illness and different health problems. It provides reliable information about each illness; <www.dipex.org>.

The HEALTH Network Group The UK Higher Education Academy Learning and Teaching in Health Network Group consists of the relevant subject centres who work closely together to support the health constituency. The Subject Centres for Health Sciences & Practice and Medicine, Dentistry & Veterinary Medicine have a single Advisory Board which has steered the work of the two Centres since 2006. Their common mission is to work together with educators, communities and organizations to promote and enhance student learning in the health-related disciplines; <http://www.heacademy.ac.uk/health/home>.

InterED The International Association for Interprofessional Education and Collaborative Practice is a collective voice and a forum for mutual exchange. InterEd's aim is to promote and advance scholarship and inform policy in interprofessional education and collaborative practice worldwide, in partnership with others; <http://www.health disciplines.ubc.ca/intered>.

JIC The *Journal of Interprofessional Care* promotes collaboration in education, practice and research worldwide. It is published by Informa Ltd, and the joint editors-in-chief are Hugh Barr and Fiona Ross; <http://www.tandf.co.uk/journals/titles/13561820.asp>.

NaHSSA National Health Sciences Students' Association of Canada & L'Association des Étudiants des Sciences de la Santé du Canada is a diverse network of eighteen university-based student chapters, which seeks to address the unmet need of actively involving Canada's health and human service students in interprofessional education, while promoting the attitudes, skills and behaviours necessary to provide collaborative patient-centred care; <http://www.nahssa.ca>.

NIPNET Nordic Interprofessional Network, a learning network to foster interprofessional collaboration in education, practice and research, primarily for Nordic educators, practitioners and researchers in the fields of health. It aims to explore the theories and evidence base of interprofessional collaboration, develops approaches, methods and evaluations of interprofessional learning and practice, stimulates exchange of ideas and experiences between countries, and fosters links with similar networks; <http://www.nipnet.org>.

The Network: TUFH The Network: Towards Unity for Health is a global association of individuals, groups, institutions and organizations committed to improving and maintaining health in the communities they have a mandate to serve. Its Interprofessional

Education Task Force has a position paper on interprofessional education; <http://www.the-network.org> and <http://www.the-networktufh.org>.

The Patient and Carer Network advises the Royal College of Physicians and enables professional bodies to take account of patient and carer views.

Appointments to this network are organized by the medical professional body and advertised in a variety of ways. Someone applying to join it is treated rather like someone applying for a job. Candidates submit information about themselves and references are sought. While it is important for professional bodies to take account of patient and carer views, successful applicants could feel it is similar to taking an unpaid job; <http://www.rcplondon.ac.uk/college/PIU/piu_pcn.asp>.

UKISN is the United Kingdom Interprofessional Students Network supported by CAIPE and Birmingham City University. Inaugurated in 2007, it seeks to support the collaboration of learners, students' interprofessional learning and their transition to practice. It can be contacted via <www.caipe.org.uk>.

References

Anning, A., Cottrell, D., Frost, N., Green, J. and Robinson, M. (2006) *Developing Multiprofessional Teamwork for Integrated Children's Services.* Buckingham: Open University Press.

Arnstein, S. (1969) A Ladder of Citizen Participation, *Journal of the American Institute of Planners* 35/4: 216–24.

Banks, S. (2006) Ethics and Values in Social Work, 3rd edn. Hampshire: Palgrave Macmillan.

Barnardo's (1998) Whose Daughter Next? Children Abused through Prostitution, London: Barnado's.

Barnett, R. and Griffen, A. (1997) *The End of Knowledge in Higher Education.* Institute of Education Series. London: Cassell.

BBC (2005) Expert patient programme investigation; programme and downloadable transcript available at: <http://www.bbc.co.uk/radio4/science/expertpatient.shtml>; accessed 8 January 2008.

Belbin Associates (2007) *Belbin Team Role Descriptions.* Cambridge: Belbin Associates <http://www.belbin.com/belbin-team-roles.htm>; accessed 26 June 2007.

Blom-Cooper, L. (1995) *The Falling Shadow.* London: Gerald Duckworth and Co Ltd.

British Medical Journal Editorial (2004) The Patient's Journey: Travelling through Life with a Chronic Illness, *British Medical Journal* 329: 582–3; <http://www.doi:10.1136/bmj.329.7466.582>.

Brown, G. W. and Harris, T. O. (1978) Social Origins of Depression: A Study of Psychiatric Disorder in Women. London: Tavistock.

Brown, H. (1999) Abuse of People with Learning Difficulties, in Stanley, N., Manthorpe, J., Penhale, B., (eds), *Institutional Abuse : Perspectives across the Life Course.* London: Routledge.

Buber, M. (1958) I and Thou, translated by Ronald Gregor Smith. New York: Charles Scribner's Sons.

Burnard, P. (1997) *Effective Communication Skills for Health Professionals,* 2nd edn. Cheltenham: Nelson Thornes.

Carers UK (2001) *How Do I get Help? Your Guide to a Carer's Assessment.* London: Carers UK; available at: <http://www.carersuk.org/Information/Helpwithcaring/Carersassessmentguide>.

Carr, S., (2004) Has Service Users Participation Made a Difference to Social Care Services? London: Social Care Institute for Excellence.

Children Act (2004) London: The Stationery Office; and also available from <www.direct.gov.uk>.

Children's Workforce Development Council (2007) *Common Assessment Framework for Children and Young People: Practitioners' Guide.* Leeds: Children's Workforce Development Council.

Clarke, Monica (2008) The Family Carer as Part of the Interprofessional Team, *CAIPE Bulletin Issue* (29 January). London: Centre for the Advancement of Education (CAIPE); available at: <http://www.caipe.org.uk.

Collins R. (1990) Changing conceptions in the sociology of the professions, in Torstendahl, R. and Burrage, M. (eds), The Formation of Professions: Knowledge, State and Strategy. London: Sage.

Coulter, A., Entwistle, V. and Gilbert, D. (1999) Sharing Decisions with Patients: Is the Information Good Enough? *British Medical Journal* 318: 318–22.

Crime and Disorder Act (1998) London: The Stationery Office; and also available from <http://www.opsi.gov.uk/acts/acts1998/ukpga_19980037_en_1>.

Data Protection Act (1998) London: The Stationery Office; and also available from <http://www.opsi.gov.uk/Acts/Acts1998/ukpga_19980029_en_1>.

Department for Children, Schools and Families (2005) *Better Information Sharing in Practice.* London: Department for Children, Schools and Families; and also available at: <www.everychildmatters.gov.uk/resources-and-practice/search/EP00082>.

Department for Education and Skills (2003) *Every Child Matters – Early Intervention and Effective Protection,* Green Paper. London: HMSO.

Department for Education and Skills (2004) *Five Year Strategy for Children and Learners,* London: Department for Education and Skills.

Department for Education and Skills (2007) Children's Workforce Strategy Update – Spring 2007 Building a World-class Workforce for Children, Young People and Families. London: Department for Education and Skills.

Department for Education and Skills (2004) *Every Child Matters: Change for Children.* London: HMSO.

Department of Health and the Home Office (2000) No Secrets: Guidance on Developing and Implementing Multi-agency Policies and Procedures to Protect Vulnerable Adults from Abuse. London: Department of Health.

Department of Health (2002) Growing Capacity: A New Role for External Healthcare Providers in England. London: Department of Health.

Department of Health and Farrell, C. (2004) *Patient and Public Involvement: The Evidence for Policy Implementation.* London: Department of Health.

Department of Health (2005a) Independence, *Well-being and Choice: Our Vision for the Future of Social Care for Adults in England,* Green Paper. London: Department of Health.

Department of Health (2005b) *The Kerr/Haslam Inquiry*. London: The Stationery Office; and also available at: <http://www.dh.gov.uk/en/Publicationsandstatistics/Publications/PublicationsPolicyAndGuidance/DH_4115349>.

Department of Health, Policy and Strategy Directorate (2006) *Health Reform in England: Update & Commissioning Framework*. London: Department of Health.

Disability Discrimination Acts (1995 and 2005) London: The Stationery Office; and also available at: <www.direct.gov.uk>.

Doncaster Council, Community and Carers Development Team (2006) Review of Adult Social Care Practice in Relation to Carers' Assessments. Doncaster: Community and Carers Development Team.

Duvvery, N., Grown, C., and Redner, J. (2004) *The Cost of Intimate Partner Violence (IPV) at the Household and Community Level*. Washington, DC: International Centre for Research on Women; and available at: <http://icrw.org/docs/2004_paper_costingviolence.pdf>.

Equal Treatment in Employment and Occupation Directive (2000) Council Directive 2000/78/EC. Brussels: Official Journal of the Europe Communities.

Every Child Matters (2008a) Government website. Available at: <http://www.everychildmatters.gov.uk/participation/faq>; accessed 6 January 2008.

Every Child Matters (2008b) *Learning to Listen: Core Principles for the Involvement of Children and Young People*. Available at: <http://www.everychildmatters.gov.uk/_files/1F85704C1D67D71E30186FEBCEDED6D6.pdf>; accessed 6 January 2008.

Fernando S. (ed) (1995) Mental Health in a Multi-ethnic Society: A Multi-disciplinary Handbook, London: Routledge.

Francis, G. and Hogg, D. (2006) Radiographer Prescribing: Enhancing Seamless Care in Oncology, *Radiography* 12/1: 3–5.

Freeth, D. (2007) *Interprofessional Education: Understanding Medical Education*. Edinburgh: Association for the Study of Medical Education.

Freeth, D., Hammick, M., Reeves, S., Koppel, I. and Barr, H. (2005) *Effective Interprofessional Education: Development, Delivery and Evaluation*. Oxford: Blackwell.

Freidson, E. (1970a) Profession of Medicine – A Study of the Sociology of Applied Knowledge. Chicago, IL: University of Chicago Press.

Freidson, E. (1970b) Professional Dominance – The Social Structure of Medical Care. New York: Atherton Press.

Freidson, E. (1994) Professionalism Reborn: Theory, Prophecy and Policy. Cambridge: Polity.

Freidson, E. (2001) *Professionalism: The Third Logic*. Cambridge: Polity.

Giddens, A. (2006) *Sociology*, 5th edn. Cambridge: Polity.

Gillies, B., Simpson, M. and Walker, L. (2004) *Learning for Effective and Ethical Practice: Opportunities for Inter-professional Learning – A Literature Review*. Dundee: Scottish Institute for Excellence in Social Work Education.

Goleman, D. (1997) *Emotional Intelligence*. London: Bloomsbury.

Hammick M., Freeth, D., Koppel, I., Reeves, S. and Barr, H. (2007) A Best Evidence Systematic Review of Interprofessional Education, BEME Guide No. 9, *Medical Teacher* 29/8: 735–51.

Hammick, M., Olckers, L. and Campion-Smith, C. (2009) Learning in Interprofessional Teams, *Association of Medical Educators in Europe Guide*. Dundee: Association of Medical Educators in Europe.

Haq, K. (2006) *The Kerr/Haslam Inquiry: The Women's Story, Witness*. Available at: <www.witnessagainstabuse.org.uk>.

Harper, Z. and Scott, S. (2005) *Meeting the Needs of Sexually Exploited Young People in London*. London: Barnardo's; available at: <www.Barnardos.org.uk>.

Hart, J. T. (1971) The Inverse Care Law, *The Lancet* 1/7696 (27 February): 405–12.

Healthcare Commission (2005) *The National Audit of Violence (2003–2005) Final Report*, London: Healthcare Commission; available from: <http://www.healthcarecommission.org.uk/db/documents/04017451.pdf>.

HM Government (2006) *Information Sharing: Practitioners' Guide*. London: Department for Education and Skills; and also available at: <www.everychildmatters.gov.uk/_files/ACB1BA35C20D4C42A1FE6F9133A7C614.pdf >.

Holland, R., Battersby, J., Harvey, I., Lenaghan, E., Smith, J. and Hay, L. (2005) Systematic Review of Multidisciplinary Interventions in Heart Failure, *Heart: British Medical Journal* 91: 899–906.

Hope, R. (2004) The Ten Essential Shared Capabilities – A Framework for the Whole of the Mental Health Workforce. London: NIMHE/SCMH Joint Workforce Support Unit.

Human Rights Act (1998) London: The Stationery Office; and also available at: <www.direct.gov.uk>.

Intercollegiate Stroke Working Party (2004) *National Clinical Guidelines for Stroke*, 2nd edn. London: Royal College of Physicians of London; 3rd edn of these guidelines is now available.

Jaques, D. and Salmon, G. (2007) *Learning in Groups*, 4th edn. London and New York: Routledge.

Jha, V., Bekker, H. L., Duffy, S. and Roberts, T. E. (2007) A Systematic Review of Studies Assessing and Facilitating Attitudes towards Professionalism in Medicine, *Medical Education* 41: 822–9.

Katzenbach, J. R. and Smith, D. K. (1993) *The Wisdom of Teams: Creating the High-Performance Organisation*. Boston: Harvard Business School.

Keating, F. (1998) *Supporting People Not Labels: Guidelines for Good Practice in the Fanon Trust*. Canterbury, Kent: Tizard Centre, University of Kent.

Kennedy, I., Howard, R., Jarman, B. and Maclean, M. (2001) Learning from Bristol: The Report of the Public Inquiry into Children's Heart Surgery at the Bristol Royal Infirmary 1984–1995. Command Paper CM 5207; and available at: <www.bristol-inquiry.org.uk/index.htm>.

Laming, Lord (2003) *Report of the Victoria Climbié Inquiry*, presented to the Secretary of State for Health and the Secretary for the Home Department; available at: <http://www.victoria-climbie-inquiry.org.uk/finreport/titlepages.htm>.

Langgartner, M., Langgartner, I. and Drlicek, M. (2005) The Patient's Journey: Multiple Sclerosis, *British Medical Journal* 330: 885–8; <http://www.doi:10.1136/bmj.330.7496.885>.

Lavender, R. and Walker, R. (2003) Simplifying the Client Journey for Females with Urinary Incontinence, *Royal Society of Medicine Bulletin* 4/2: 6–9; available at: <www.clinical-governance.com>.

Leicht, K. T. and Fennel, M. L. (2001) *Professional Work: A Sociological Approach*. Oxford: Blackwell.

Levin, E. (2004) *Involving Service Users and Carers in Social Work Education*. London: Social Care Institute for Excellence.

Liabo, K., Bolton, A., Copperman, J., Curtis, K., Downie, A. and Palmer, T. (2000) *The Sexual Exploitation of Children and Young People in Lambeth, Southwark and Lewisham*. London: Barnardo's.

Lipsett, A. (2006) You'll Go Far if You Can Show Some Emotion. *Times Higher Education Supplement* (24 November); available at: <www.timeshighereducation.co.uk/issueIndex.asp?issueCode=370>; accessed November 2008.

McCabe, A., Lowndes, V. and Skelcher, C. (1997) *Partnerships and Networks: An Evaluation and Development Manual*. York: Joseph Rowntree Foundation.

Macdonald, K. M. (1995) *The Sociology of the Professions*. London: Sage.

McGill, I. and Brockbank, A. (2004) *The Action Learning Handbook*. London: Routledge-Falmer.

McKenna, E (2000) *Business Psychology and Organisational Behaviour: A Student Handbook*, 3rd edn. East Sussex: Psychology Press; part of the Taylor Francis Group.

Malone, D., Newron-Howes, G., Simmonds, S., Marriot, S. and Tyrer, P. (2007) *Community Mental Health Teams (CMHTs) for People with Severe Mental Illnesses and Disordered Personality*. Oxford: Cochrane Library, Issue 3.

Mayer, J. D. and Salovey, P. (1997) What is Emotional Intelligence?, in P. Salovey and D. Sluyter (eds), *Emotional Development and Emotional Intelligence: Educational Applications*. New York: Basic Books, pp. 3–31.

Meads, G. and Ashcroft, J. (eds) (2005) The Case for Interprofessional Collaboration in Health and Social Care. Oxford: Blackwell.

Meads, G. and Barr, H. (2005) Learning Together, in G. Meads and J. Ashcroft (eds), *The Case for Interprofessional Collaboration in Health and Social Care*. Oxford: Blackwell.

Mental Capacity Act (2005) London: The Stationery Office; and also available at: <www.direct.gov.uk>.

Mental Welfare Commission for Scotland (2006) *Carers and*

Confidentiality: Developing Effective Relationships between Practitioners and Carers. Edinburgh: Mental Welfare Commission for Scotland.

National Institute for Clinical Excellence (2004) *Guidance for Cancer Services: Improving Supportive and Palliative Care for Adults with Cancer*. London: National Institute for Clinical Excellence.

Neill, M., Hayward, K. S. and Peterson, T. (2007) Students' Perceptions of the Interprofessional Team in Practice through the Application of Servant Leadership Principles, *Journal of Interprofessional Care* 21/4: 425–32.

Parker, J. and Bradley, G. (2003) Social Work Practice: Assessment, Planning, Intervention and Review. Exeter: Learning Matters.

Parker, C. and McCulloch, A. (1999) Key Issues from Homicide Inquiries – an Analysis Carried out for MIND. London: MIND.

Parrott, L., Jacobs, G., and Roberts, D. (2008) SCIE Research briefing 23: *Stress and Resilience Factors in Parents with Mental Health Problems and Their Children*; downloadable as a pfd at: <www.scie.org.uk>.

Payne, M. (1997) *Modern Social Work Theory*, 2nd edn. New York: Palgrave.

Pierson, J. (2002) *Tackling Social Exclusion*. Abingdon: Routledge.

Pollock, A. (2004) *NHS plc*. London: Verso.

Pritchard, A. (2005) Ways of Learning, Learning Theories and Learning Styles in the Classroom. London: David Fulton Publishers Ltd.

Quality Assurance Agency for Higher Education for England (undated) *Statement of Common Purpose for Subject Benchmark Statements for the Health and Social Care Professions*. Bristol: Quality Assurance Agency for Higher Education for England.

Race Relations Act (1976) London: The Stationery Office; and also available at: <www.direct.gov.uk>.

Ritchie, J., Dick, D. and Lingham, R. (1994) *Report of the Inquiry into the Care and Treatment of Christopher Clunis*. London: The Stationery Office.

Rose, D. (2001) Users' Voices: The Perspectives of Mental Health Service Users on Community and Hospital Care. London: Sainsbury Centre for Mental Health.

Royal College of Psychiatrists (1996) Report of the Confidential Inquiry into Homicides and Suicides by Mentally Disordered Offenders. London: Royal College of Psychiatrists.

Seale, C. and Pattison, S. (1994) *Medical Knowledge: Doubt and Certainty*, Milton Keynes: Open University Press.

Sex Discrimination Act (1975) London: The Stationery Office; and also available at: <www.direct.gov.uk>.

Silverblatt, H. and Seeger, K (2007) Enhancing Community-University Partnerships in a Rural State, *The Network Towards Unity for Health Newsletter* 26/2: <http://www.the-networktufh.org/publications_resources/newsletterdetail.asp?id=14&tt=Newsletter%0D%0A&t=The+Newsletters+(full+text)>; accessed 29 August 2008.

Simmonds, S., Coid, J., Philip, J., Marriott, S. and Tyrer, P. (2001) Community Mental Health Team Management in Severe Mental Illness: A Systematic Review, *The British Journal of Psychiatry* 178: 497–502.

Social Care Institute for Excellence (2006) *Practice Guide 2: Assessing the Mental Health Needs of Older People*. Available from: <http://www.scie.org.uk/publications/practiceguides/practiceguide02>.

Soubhi, H. (2007) The Greatest Challenge of Interprofessional Education, *Newsletter, The Network: Towards Unity For Health* 26/2; available at: < www.the-networktufh.org/download.asp?file=NL022007.pdf>.

Spears, L. C. and Lawrence, M. (eds) (2002) Insights on Leadership: Service, Stewardship, Spirit, and Servant Leadership. Toronto: John Wiley and Sons.

Stewart, M. (2001) Towards a Global Definition of Patient Centred Care, *British Medical Journal* 322: 444–5.

Tait L. & Shah S. (2007) Partnership working: a policy with promise for mental healthcare, *Advances in Psychiatric Treatment* 13:261-271.

Taylor, I., Sharland, E., Sebbia, J. and Leriche, P. (2006) *The Learning, Teaching and Assessment of Partnership Working in Social Work Education.* London: Social Care Institute for Excellence.

Tew, J. (2005) *Social Perspectives in Mental Health.* London: Jessica Kingsley.

Thomson, K. (1998) *Emotional Capital.* Oxford: Capstone Publishing Ltd.

The Times (2007) The Vitamin That May Give Timothy His Childhood Back (20 March). Available at: <http://www.timesonline.co.uk/tol/news/uk/health/article1539593.ec>.

Tope, R., Thomas, E. and Jones, M. E. (2008) Report to Walsall Teaching Primary Care Trust on Low Birth Weight Babies Research Project Developing a Strategy. Wales: HERC Associates.

Townsend, P., Davidson, N. and Whitehead, M. (eds) (1992) *Inequalities in Health: The Black Report, The Health Divide,* 2nd edn. Harmondworth: Penguin.

Townsley, Ruth and Goodwin, Julian (2003) *All About Feeling Down.* Bristol: Generate organization, Norah Fry Research Centre, University of Bristol; available at: <http://www.learningdisabilities.org.uk>.

Tuckman, B. W. (1965) Developmental Sequence in Small Groups, *Psychological Bulletin* 63: 384–99.

User Focused Monitoring Team (2000) *User Focused Monitoring of Mental Health Service in Huntingdonshire.* London: Sainsbury Centre for Mental Health.

Ward, J. (1993) *Violence Against People with Serious Mental Health Problems.* Toronto: Canadian Mental Health Association.

West, M. (2004) Effective Teamwork, Practical Lessons from Organisational Research, 2nd edn. Oxford: Blackwell.

Wicks, E. (2007) A Patient's Journey Cystic Fibrosis, *British Medical*

Journal 334: 1270–1; available at: <http://www.bmj.com/cgi/
content/full/334/7606/0> (accessed 9 September 2008).

Wikipedia (2008) *Emotional Intelligence (EI)*. Available at: <http://
en.wikipedia.org/wiki/Emotional_intelligence>; accessed 15
January 2008.

Wilmott, S. (1995) Professional Values and Inter-professional
Dialogue, *Journal of Interprofessional Care* 9/3: 257–66.

Winkler, F. (1994) Transferring Power in Health Care, in B. Davey,
A. Gray and C. Seale (eds), *Health and Disease: A Reader*, 2nd edn.
Buckingham: Open University Press.

World Health Organisation Study Group on Multiprofessional
Education for Health Personnel (1987) *Learning Together to Work
Together for Health*. Geneva: World Health Organisation.

World Health Organisation (2008) *Palliative Care*. Geneva: World
Health Organisation; and available at: http://www.who.int/cancer/
palliative/en/>; accessed 27 August 2008.

World Health Organisation Study Group on Interprofessional
Education and Collaborative Practice (forthcoming) *World Health
Organisation Framework for Action on Interprofessional Education and
Collaborative Practice*. Geneva: World Health Organisation.

Index